BREAKING THE GLASS CEILING

The Stories of Three Caribbean Nurses

Jocelyn Hezekiah

Order this book online at www.trafford.com/03-1895
or email orders@trafford.com

Most Trafford titles are also available at major online book retailers.

© Copyright 2003 Jocelyn Hezekiah

All rights reserved. No part of this publication may be reproduced, stored in a retrieval system, or transmitted, in any form or by any means, electronic, mechanical, photocopying, recording, or otherwise, without the written prior permission of the author.

First printing: University of the West Indies Press Biography Series, Published 2001

Cover and book design by Paul Butts.

Note for Librarians: A cataloguing record for this book is available from Library and Archives Canada at www.collectionscanada.ca/amicus/index-e.html

Printed in Victoria, BC, Canada.

ISBN: 978-1-4120-1517-2

We at Trafford believe that it is the responsibility of us all, as both individuals and corporations, to make choices that are environmentally and socially sound. You, in turn, are supporting this responsible conduct each time you purchase a Trafford book, or make use of our publishing services. To find out how you are helping, please visit www.trafford.com/responsiblepublishing.html

Our mission is to efficiently provide the world's finest, most comprehensive book publishing service, enabling every author to experience success. To find out how to publish your book, your way, and have it available worldwide, visit us online at www.trafford.com/10510

Trafford
PUBLISHING

www.trafford.com

North America & international
toll-free: 1 888 232 4444 (USA & Canada)
phone: 250 383 6864 ♦ fax: 250 383 6804
email: info@trafford.com

The United Kingdom & Europe
phone: +44 (0)1865 722 113 ♦ local rate: 0845 230 9601
facsimile: +44 (0)1865 722 868 ♦ email: info.uk@trafford.com

10 9 8 7 6 5 4

Contents

List of Illustrations *vi*

Foreword *viii*

Preface and Acknowledgements *x*

Introduction *xiii*

Abbreviations *xix*

PART I: NITA BARROW

Chapter One
Laying the Groundwork: Service and Activism *3*

Chapter Two
Reaching the Pinnacle *34*

PART II: BERENICE DOLLY

Chapter Three
A Woman of Action *73*

Chapter Four
Developing the Nursing Profession *97*

PART III: MARY JANE SEIVWRIGHT

Chapter Five
Beating the Odds *139*

Chapter Six
An Extraordinary Woman *162*

Conclusion *204*

Bibliography *210*

Index *215*

Illustrations

1.1	Formal portrait of Dame Nita Barrow, 1993 / *2*	
1.2	On the grounds of University of Toronto, 1944 / *19*	
1.3	Nita Barrow with Ivy Lawrence, Wilma Cameron and Eugenia Charles, Toronto, 1944 / *20*	
1.4	Nita Barrow and friends, University of Toronto, 1944 / *21*	
1.5	Battered, weather-beaten suitcase, Jamaica, 1945 / *25*	
1.6	President of the Nurses' Association of Jamaica, 1946–48 / *29*	
1.7	Presidents of the Nurses' Association of Jamaica, 1946–56 / *30*	
2.1	Caribbean Nurses' Organization Meeting, 1968 / *38*	
2.2	Dame Nita mixing with the crowds, Barbados, 1995 / *64*	
2.3	Bust of Dame Nita / *66*	
3.1	Ben Dolly, Pointe-à-Pierre, Trinidad, 1996 / *72*	
3.2	Ben Dolly and family, Maraval, Trinidad, 1996 / *83*	
3.3	President of Soroptimists International of Trinidad and Tobago, 1976 / *91*	
4.1	Ben Dolly, prior to entry into nursing, 1936 / *102*	
4.2	Nursing Council Building, 1979 / *114*	
4.3	Plaque, Dolly-Hargreaves Building, 1979 / *115*	
4.4	Admission to the International Council of Nurses, Brazil, 1953 / *118*	
4.5	Sightseeing, International Council of Nurses' congress, Rome, 1957 / 119	
4.6	Caribbean nurses after church service, Caribbean Nurses' Organization biennial conference, 1980 / *123*	

Illustrations

4.7	Relaxing at the Caribbean Nurses' Organization thirteenth biennial conference, Bahamas, 1982 / *124*
4.8	After the church service, Caribbean Nurses' Organization thirteenth biennial conference, Bahamas, 1982 / *125*
4.9	Nurses' Week, Methodist Church, Port of Spain, Trinidad, 1979 / *131*
4.10	Second quadrennial health seminar, 1987 / *133*
4.11	Working behind the scenes, biennial general meeting, 1994 / *134*
5.1	Mary Jane Seivwright, president of the Nurses' Association of Jamaica / *138*
5.2	Summer school, Kingston, Jamaica, 1969 / *157*
5.3	Fourteenth quadrennial congress, International Council of Nurses, Montreal, Canada, 1969 / *159*
5.4	Delegates to the Commonwealth nursing seminar, Barbados, 1970 / *160*
6.1	Mary with Enid Lawrence, Nurse Practitioner Programme, Jamaica, 1982 / *177*
6.2	Nursing Education Seminar, Kingston, Jamaica, 1973 / *183*
6.3	Jamaican delegation, International Council of Nurses, Korea, 1989 / *184*
6.4	Socializing at the forty-fifth annual general meeting of the Nurses' Association of Jamaica, Ocho Rios, 1991 / *187*
6.5	Unveiling plaque in the boardroom, Nurses' Association of Jamaica, Kingston, 1995 / *187*
6.6	With past presidents and honoured nurses, Nurses' Association of Jamaica, Kingston, 1995 / *189*
6.7	With Japanese Nursing Association, International Council of Nurses, Tokyo, Japan, 1977 / *197*
6.8	At the naming ceremony, Mona, Jamaica, 1997 / *198*
6.9	Mary Jane Seivwright Building, Mona, Jamaica, 1997 / *199*

Foreword

Jocelyn Hezekiah's book is long overdue. Very little has been written about the mammoth contribution made by Caribbean nurse leaders either in their own country or internationally. This book will close that gap to a great extent. It is the first really comprehensive treatise of three fascinating nurses of the Caribbean. It describes vividly the lives and times of the distinguished nurse leaders – Dame Nita Barrow from Barbados, Berenice Dolly from Trinidad, and Dr Mary Seivwright from Jamaica.

My long professional journey with these three dynamic nurse leaders began in 1962, on the day I completed my oral examination for a doctoral degree. On completion of the doctoral examination, it was the custom of Teachers' College, Columbia University, to celebrate by gathering for coffee in the cafeteria with faculty and other doctoral students. I was enjoying my success when a beautiful dark-skinned woman approached me at the faculty table and said, "I'm Nita Barrow and I would like to talk with you." Then, later, she said, "I would like you to come to the Caribbean and conduct a survey of our schools of nursing like you did in Canada." That encounter changed my whole life and, in this context, influenced the health services of the Caribbean as did the Canadian survey conducted in Canada. Nita later became a dynamic force in the health and social sectors in the Caribbean and globally, and our friendship endured throughout her lifetime.

I recall with warmth and gratitude the presence and contribution of Berenice Dolly as a member of the Board of Review for the Survey of Schools of Nursing in the Caribbean area in 1966, and at subsequent sessions of groups related to the project. Participating as a member of the Board of Review for the project was a difficult task in many respects. It required reading, analysing and reporting on hundreds of pages of documentation for the surveys of twenty-three schools of nursing in fourteen countries and territories. For each school, board members examined the philosophy and objectives, the organization and administration, the instructional personnel, the student services, the curriculum, the evaluation process, the library, the setting for the educational programme, and the physical facilities. Ben was outstanding at these meetings. Visiting health and educational facilities with Ben was a joy and a valuable experience. On every occasion, the faculty and tutor in each setting welcomed her with both respect and affection. Nowhere in the entire Caribbean had we viewed such interesting displays of curriculum content and recreational programmes. It was evident that she worked hard to achieve her objectives not only related to nursing but to the community at large. Our encounters convinced me that she was a modern day activist putting others before self.

I met Mary Seivwright in many venues throughout the Caribbean. In our meetings on nursing education, Mary was formidable. She stood out as a dynamic visionary with practical solutions. Events have confirmed that she was an extraordinary woman. Her achievements attest to her greatness and leadership throughout the region and in the world at large. I remember her as an outstanding participant at the PAHO/WHO Nursing Education seminar in 1971 and at other meetings.

These three nurses were well known to Jocelyn Hezekiah. However, this did not detract from her ability to write an objective scholarly account of their outstanding contributions to the health and welfare of the citizens of the region. She is to be commended for her foresight in selecting these particular nursing leaders. This account of their lives will inspire a new generation of health professionals.

The comprehensiveness of *Breaking the Glass Ceiling* provides readers both in the health services and other disciplines with a unique perspective of the health services in the Caribbean, offering a view of how these three nurse leaders from different islands have made a difference and 'moved the world'. The author has blended in facts and analysis with a keen eye for their significance, and has brought to life the three women with warmth, humanity and clarity. This book is distinctly illuminating and can deepen, widen, refine and enrich our knowledge of nursing and health services in the Caribbean.

Helen Mussallem

Preface and Acknowledgements

The history of nursing and those who shaped the profession and health care has been an interest of mine for as long as I can remember. For many years, I taught courses in the history of nursing to nursing students in Canada. Consequently, within recent years, with the formation of history of nursing associations, I became a member of the Ontario, Canadian and American history of nursing associations. I recall vividly at one of the very early conferences in Canada being the only person of colour, and the last presenter, speaking about the contributions of black nurses from a small developing nation. This was an offshoot of my doctoral dissertation which addressed the development of nursing education in Trinidad and Tobago from 1956 to 1986. All the other papers presented concerned the contributions of nurses, nursing religious (nuns), and leaders from the European world. It may have been coincidental that the first speaker was from Great Britain, the other presenters were from the white Canadian world and I, as the last presenter, spoke about the West Indies. I commented 'tongue in cheek' that it seemed that the colonial relationship was still in evidence at this conference even in 1986.

Since I felt strongly that the contributions and accomplishments of Caribbean nurses were not recognized or documented, it was logical that I would embark upon this project. The opportunity to pursue this goal came in the form of a six-month sabbatical, from January to June 1996, from McMaster University in Hamilton, Ontario. I documented the achievements and lived experiences of three Caribbean nursing leaders in the development of nursing and health care in the Caribbean and the wider world during the colonial and postcolonial era, 1940–

1990. I chose that period as it covered the late colonial era, about two decades prior to independence of many of the islands, and two to three decades into the postcolonial period. The late colonial and early postcolonial decades were a watershed in Caribbean history as the struggle for indigenous leadership in all areas of West Indian society was being fought.

But equally important was the fact that many of the nurses who provided leadership at that time had died or were ageing and it was critical for me to capture their stories and see their experiences from their vantage point. I do not lay claim that this is a definitive historical or feminist work but rather that it is a narrative of the lives of these women, albeit not as comprehensive as it could be. I seek merely to begin the journey and it behoves others to continue the task. Specifically, I documented their contributions and examined from a feminist and colonialist perspective the political, social and economic context prior to and during their personal and professional development. The factors and influences that contributed to or hindered their development were explored, and I identified and located some of the other nursing leaders of Caribbean heritage in the West Indies. The latter could provide a preliminary database for future researchers.

Because of time and financial constraints, I focused on the contributions of three eminent and ageing nursing leaders in three Caribbean islands: Dame Nita Barrow from Barbados, Berenice Dolly from Trinidad, and Dr Mary Seivwright from Jamaica. Their choice was obvious as they are known throughout the Caribbean and internationally. I must, however, acknowledge my own personal bias as I knew these three women and had encountered them frequently in my professional life. I had kept in touch with them over the years and have always had a high regard and great admiration for them. These factors did influence my choice. In addition, I had been privileged to have Dame Nita as the external advisor for my doctoral dissertation in Alberta, Canada, many years ago.

I envisioned this project as having many useful outcomes. It could benefit women in general and visible minority women in particular because a small part of women's history will be written for present and future generations. Knowledge will be provided that could help to give Caribbean nurses a feeling of belonging and identification and encourage group pride. Further, it would yield valuable and important contributions to a severely underdeveloped area in the history of international nursing and health care. Finally, it would allow Caribbean nurses to examine their past in order to understand their present professional development and, with that knowledge, plan future endeavours.

Preface and Acknowledgements

I am deeply indebted to a number of people and institutions. This book could not have become a reality without them, in particular, the Arts Council, the Social Sciences and Humanities Research Council, for providing me with a grant that allowed me to visit the Caribbean to undertake this project, and the Nurses' Association of Jamaica, and the Trinidad and Tobago Registered Nurses' Association for opening their libraries to me. I owe a debt of gratitude to Sir Kenneth Standard not only for his willingness to be interviewed but also for providing me with archival documents from the Department of Social and Preventive Medicine, University of the West Indies, Mona. I am most grateful for the help, encouragement and support from many friends, colleagues and relatives. Particular mention is due to Eng Ming Chong and my niece Gael Garland, for their meticulous editing of my manuscript. Special thanks to Barb Carpio and Jessie Mantle for their insightful suggestions and constructive criticism of the manuscript. My greatest debt of gratitude is due to the many men and women in St Kitts, Nevis, Barbados, Trinidad and Jamaica who so willingly allowed me to interview them. The generosity of all those in the islands who opened their homes to me during my sojourn is deeply appreciated.

I am grateful to all who gave so unstintingly of their time to share with me their insights and their experiences with these three women, and I am privileged to have had these three women share their narratives with me. It is with much pride that I recount their stories through their own voices and those of their many colleagues, students and friends. In spite of imperfections, I hope that you will enjoy reading this book as much as I have enjoyed writing it.

Introduction

Within recent times, the role of nurses in the health care system and the influence of their unique perspective on health care reform have increasingly received attention. This is particularly evident in recorded works about pioneering British and Canadian nurses such as Florence Nightingale, Isabel Robb and Adelaide Nutting. Nursing literature is replete with documentation of the achievements and accomplishments of nursing leaders from the developed world – British, American, Canadian, European and, lately, Australian – and their impact on nursing in their own countries and internationally. This issue of leadership assumes greater significance when it involves the developing countries as nursing leadership was traditionally always provided by the dominant group from the metropolitan countries. There is a dearth of documented research about the contributions of nursing leaders to the health care system in the developing world. In terms of a multicultural and international perspective, one might well ask where, if any, are the nursing leaders of African, Asian and Caribbean heritage in the developing countries? What are their achievements? Did they become leaders during the time of European dominance? Or is it only in the postcolonial period? If there are leaders in the developing countries, why have their contributions to nursing and health care not been acknowledged and documented?

A review of the literature identified only a few books and journal articles written about nurses of colour, and it is not coincidental that the authors were of the same cultural and racial background. D.C. Hine, a black American female historian, writing about the history of black health professionals in the health care system in the United States of America examined the intersection between class, race and gender. She observed that black nurses were denied opportunities for administrative and leadership positions within their chosen profession because "such positions were considered the preserve of either black male physicians or white female administrators".[1] Just as the history of nursing assumed only white nursing history, so did books on black history exclude nursing, which is still a predominantly female profession, until M.E. Carnegie, a black American nurse historian, addressed the issue of blacks in nursing in the United States. Her recent publication briefly highlighted some of the efforts of African and Caribbean nurses. More recently, A.T. Davis examined the contributions of early black American nursing leaders. Within the past few years, nursing leadership was also examined internationally by Splane and Splane through a focused examination of chief nursing officer positions in ministries of health.[2] Of central concern was the lack of in-depth documentation about the contributions of Caribbean nurses and nursing leaders, although a few historical articles and doctoral dissertations have been written by Caribbean nurses and physicians documenting health services, health policies, and nursing education. In particular, Mary Seivwright and Syringa Marshall-Burnett from the Caribbean both focused on the contributions of Mary Seacole, one of the earliest black Jamaican nurses, who set up her own hospital for British soldiers during the Crimean War and whose work was largely ignored until recent times.[3] Clearly, the invisibility of the contributions of nurses and nursing leadership in the Caribbean to the development of the profession and health care nationally and internationally needed to be addressed. Nursing history had marginalized them too long. I believed that the voices of these women needed to be heard and their achievements and experiences written and shared with future generations.

The methodology I used was that of feminist oral history. I chose this method because we are primarily an oral society. Record keeping is not one of our strengths. In fact, trying to get documents in the islands was a daunting and difficult task. Moreover, I wanted to hear from these women their perceptions and recollections of people and events. Documenting the recollections of ageing people could be criticized since it could be argued that their accounts might not coincide with the facts. But I contend that their interpretation of facts has validity and records, where available, were used to substantiate actual events. The perceptions of these nurses are factual to the extent that we acknowledge that each of us interprets events from our own set of lenses, given the same set of data. Moreover, there are no records that purport to document systematically the contributions of Caribbean nurses.

Introduction

The form of the oral discourse was through interactive dialogue with the narrators so that issues and events that they deemed important emerged.[4] It allowed them to tell their stories in their own way. A number of potential issues and topics served as a guide to the discussion.[5] For example, I asked them to start wherever they wished. Some unforeseen limitations transpired during the conduct of this study. Dame Nita died before her oral history was completed, and Dr Mary Seivwright was indisposed at the time when I was collecting data in Jamaica so that a series of telephone dialogues was necessary, rather than face-to-face contact. Notwithstanding this, I was able to interview thirty-three colleagues in five islands (St Kitts, Nevis, Barbados, Trinidad and Jamaica) regarding these three women. Selection of these colleagues was carried out by reputation; that is, the three narrators as well as current nursing leaders suggested names from a variety of professions and disciplines, until a saturation point was achieved. The interviews were tape recorded and later transcribed.

These primary data were supplemented by archival research – official and non-official in Barbados, Trinidad and Jamaica – as well as in official documents from the Pan-American Health Organization/World Health Organization (PAHO/WHO) in Washington, DC, and libraries in Canada.

I chose to use a feminist and colonialist theoretical perspective for the exploration of political, social and economic structures of the societies prior to and during the lifetimes of these nurses in order to provide a context for their achievements and contributions. I think that this approach was most appropriate for an examination of the lives of these women who lived in both the colonial and postcolonial eras and indeed could be considered feminists, though none of them would characterize themselves as such.

Nita Barrow in Barbados, Berenice 'Ben' Dolly in Trinidad and Mary Seivwright in Jamaica were born between 1916 and 1923, during the late colonial era. Each would have a considerable impact on the status of women and the development of the nursing profession separately and later, at times, together. Unknown to each other they would enter the same profession, work relentlessly for the advancement of women and eventually, by fortunate coincidence, meet at particular points in time to work together for the betterment of nurses nationally and regionally. They all made international contributions. The late Dame Nita Barrow was the most outstanding of the three women in international stature. Mrs Ben Dolly, who served on the International Council of Nurses (ICN) for many years, is a versatile and influential leader, and Dr Mary Jane Seivwright is an internationally known, brilliant nurse.

Introduction

This book traces the lives of these three women. The first part looks at young Nita Barrow and her middle-class upbringing. She was greatly influenced by her family, especially her activist father who championed the causes of the poor and underprivileged, and whose ministry took the family to many islands, thus giving her a Caribbean identity. The various nursing positions she held in the Caribbean and her impact on the region in terms of nursing and health care are developed. Her activism and commitment to the development of women and her championship of human rights regionally and internationally, as well as her many distinguished awards, led to her appointment to one of the Caribbean's highest positions as governor general of Barbados.

The second part looks at Ben Dolly. Like Nita, Ben had a middle-class upbringing with parents who were involved in community life. The only married woman of the three nurses, Ben's manifold activities within her home and the community are explored. The influence of her family life with her husband, a physician, who facilitated her professional and social activism, is examined. Her zeal and relentless drive for the registration of nurses and membership in the ICN, and for the causes of women gave her recognition and awards nationally.

The third profile is that of Dr Mary Jane Seivwright. Mary, unlike Nita and Ben, was born of humble parentage. The key influences in her early life, her determination, her postgraduate studies in the United States, and her work as a consultant with the ICN laid the groundwork for this extraordinary woman to become the first Caribbean woman to head the first Bachelor of Science in Nursing programme at the University of the West Indies (UWI). Her crusades to get the Nurse Practitioner Programme implemented and to have the Advanced Nursing Education Unit become an established department at UWI were her passion as director of the unit. Equally important was her singular devotion to the Nurses' Association of Jamaica and the Nursing Council. Her political involvement as a senator and her many accolades and honours were only fitting for one who beat the odds and climbed the ladder of success with grit and determination.

These women share as many similarities as differences. They were bright, black women who embraced each challenge that came their way as an opportunity for growth. This growth was not for personal gain or self-aggrandizement but for the good of womankind and the nursing profession. The common distinguishing feature of these three women was their selfless devotion to service. They worked relentlessly to improve the image of nursing, the nursing profession, and the status of women. Each one did so in her unique way, and each had a deep, abiding religious faith. In the experience of the black woman, class and sex, like race, have

Introduction

never been independent or autonomous processes. From birth, the possibilities open to any woman are largely predetermined by her class and racial background, as well as by her sex. Her future will be largely determined by the interplay of various forces that impinge on each other at particular points in time.[6] This truism will become apparent as the stories of these three women depict their different approaches to their service to women in general and nursing in particular, whether in the international arena, in the Caribbean setting or in their own native land. They were outstanding role models. They rose to prominence in a society in which race, gender and class distinctions existed.

I chose the title *Breaking the Glass Ceiling*, a term coined almost two decades ago, to denote that invisible barrier that is both structural and attitudinal, and in male-dominated occupations prevents women from reaching the top. Although they did not break barriers in a male-dominated profession, where the term is more properly applied, they broke the limits that were defined for black women at that time. They defied tradition within a traditional woman's occupation. They transcended barriers of race, gender and class within a patriarchal society and did so with sustained vitality and more political awareness than most women at that time. They blazed the way for black women, and nurses in particular, to reach for the top. They were the first black women in nursing in the Caribbean to receive national and international acclaim, though not all to the same extent, and were acknowledged role models for black nurses and women in the region.

Notes

1. D.C. Hine, *Black Women in White: Racial Conflict and Cooperation in the Nursing Profession, 1890–1950* (Bloomington: Indiana University Press, 1989), xviii. Hine's book explored black American health care professionals with a focus on black nurses.
2. M.E. Carnegie, *The Path We Tread: Blacks in Nursing Worldwide 1854–1994*, 3d ed. (New York: National League for Nursing Press, 1995); A.T. Davis, *Early Black American Leaders in Nursing: Architects for Integration and Equity* (Sudbury, Mass: Jones and Bartlett, 1999); S.K. Khanna, *History of Nursing in India from 1947–1989* (Missouri: Cape Girardeau, 1991); K. Kodamer, *Nursing in Japan* (Tokyo: Nippon Kango Kyokai, Showersznner, 1977); R. Splane and V. Splane, *Chief Nursing Officer Positions in National Ministries of Health: Focal Point for Nursing Leadership* (San Francisco: The Regents, School of Nursing, University of California, San Francisco, 1994); A.B. Thoms, *Pathfinders: A History of the Progress of Colored Graduate Nurses*

(New York: Garland, 1985). These authors addressed specifically the contributions of nurses from their own cultures. Carnegie, Davis and Thoms looked at black American nurses, with an overview of the Caribbean by Carnegie in her later edition. Khanna focused on the Indian setting, while Kodamer looked at the Japanese. Splane and Splane, Canadians, examined leadership dimensions from an international perspective by focusing on the role of principal nursing officers.

3. S. Marshall-Burnett, "A Brief Reflection on the Life of Mary Seacole, 1805–1881", *Jamaican Nurse* 21, no. 2 (1981): 14–15; M.J. Seivwright, "The Florence Nightingale of Jamaica", *Jamaican Nurse* 21, no. 2 (1981): 16; L.M. Comissiong, "Health Services in the British Caribbean: 1935–1969", *Caribbean Medical Journal* 30 (1970): 40–42; E. De Verteuil, "The Urgent Need for a Medical and Health Policy for Trinidad", *Caribbean Medical Journal* 5, no. 3 (1943): 107–19; J. Grayson, "The Nurses' Association of Trinidad and Tobago" (DEd diss., Teachers' College, Columbia University, 1989); J. Hezekiah, "Post-colonial Nursing Education in Trinidad and Tobago", *Advances in Nursing Science* 12, no. 2 (1990): 28–36; J. Hezekiah, "The Development of Health Care Policies in Trinidad and Tobago: Autonomy or Domination?", *International Journal of Health Services* 19, no. 1 (1989): 79–93; J. Hezekiah, "Nursing Leadership and the Colonial Heritage", *Image: Journal of Nursing Scholarship* 20, no. 3 (1988): 155–58; P. Hay Ho Sang, "The Development of Nursing Education in Jamaica, West Indies: 1900–1975" (DEd diss., Teachers' College, Columbia University, 1984); S.M. Laurence, "The Evolution of the Trinidad Midwife", *Caribbean Medical Journal* 3, no. 4 (1941): 204–8.

4. Unless otherwise indicated, all material quoted from Dame Nita Barrow, Ben Dolly and Dr Mary Jane Seivwright comes from personal interviews with the author during the course of this research.

5. See K. Minister, "A Feminist Frame for the Oral History Interview", in *Women's Words: The Feminist Practice of Oral History*, edited by H. Gluck and D. Patai (New York: Routledge, Chapman and Hall, 1991), 27–42, where the approach to collecting data from a feminist perspective is discussed in greater detail.

6. R.E. Reddock, *Women, Labour and Struggle in Twentieth Century Trinidad and Tobago, 1898–1960* (The Hague: Institute of Social Studies, 1984), 70.

Abbreviations

ANEU	Advanced Nursing Education Unit
CMC	Christian Medical Commission
CNO	Caribbean Nurses' Organization
CNR	Council of National Representatives
DANE	Department of Advanced Nursing Education
DAWN	Development Alternatives for Women
HMSO	Her (His) Majesty's Stationery Office
HOPE	Health Opportunities for People Everywhere
ICAE	International Council of Adult Education
ICN	International Council of Nurses
IDT	Industrial Disputes Tribunal
JGTNA	Jamaica General Trained Nurses' Association
KPH	Kingston Public Hospital
MAJ	Medical Association of Jamaica
NAJ	Nurses' Association of Jamaica
NIHERST	National Institute for Higher Education, Research, Science and Technology
PAHO/WHO	Pan-American Health Organization of the World Health Organization
TNMATT	Trained Nurses and Midwives' Association of Trinidad and Tobago
TRINCAS	Trinidad Counselling and Advisory Service
TTRNA	Trinidad and Tobago Registered Nurses' Association
UCHWI	University College Hospital of the West Indies

Abbreviations

UCWI	University College of the West Indies
UN	United Nations
UNESCO	United Nations Educational, Scientific and Cultural Organization
UNIA	Universal Negro Improvement Association
UWI	University of the West Indies
WCC	World Council of Churches
WISPH	West Indies School of Public Health
YWCA	Young Women's Christian Association

PART I

Nita Barrow

If you can talk with crowds and keep your virtue
Or walk with kings – nor lose the common touch.

Rudyard Kipling

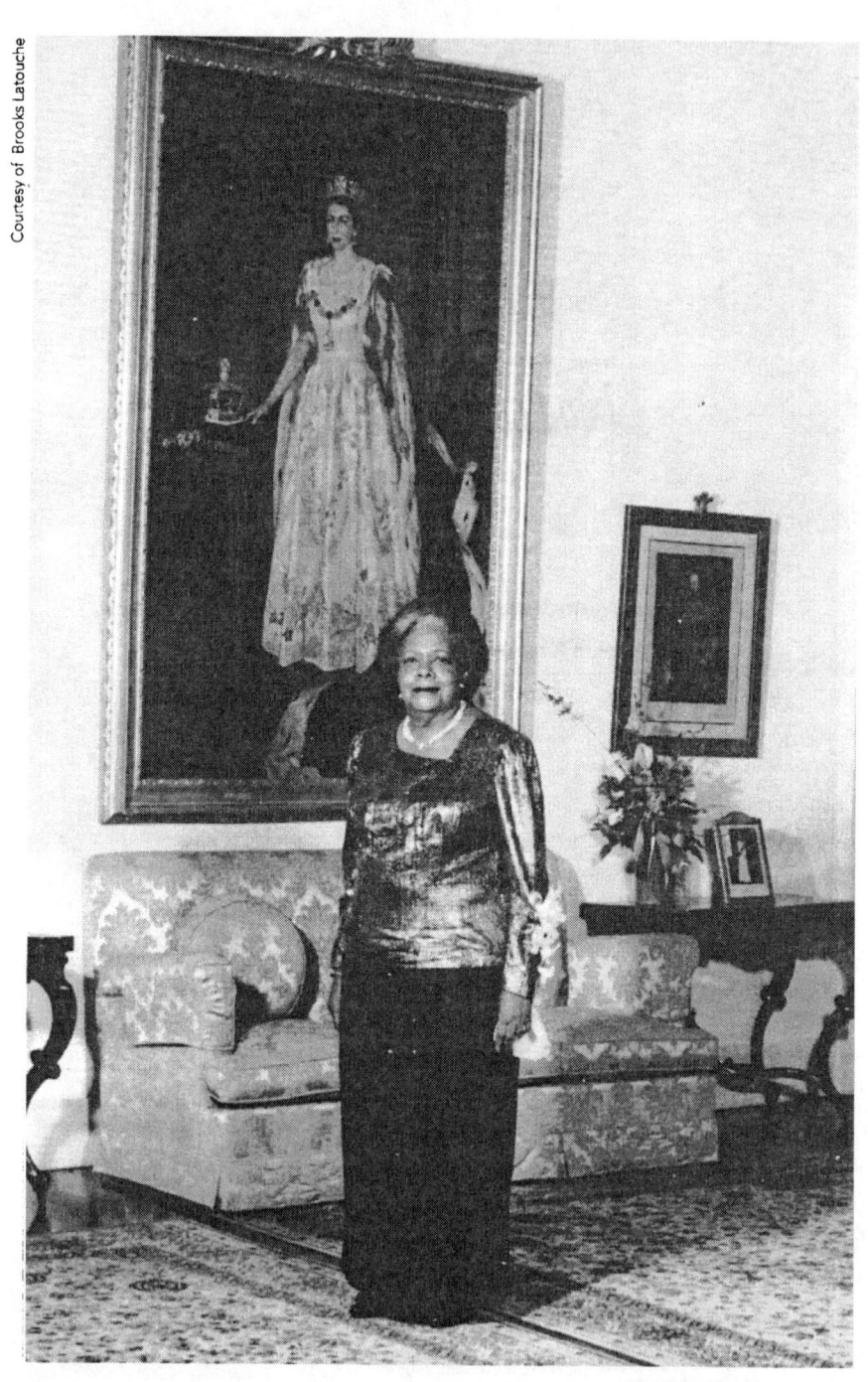

Formal portrait of Dame Nita Barrow, governor general, Government House Barbados, 1993

CHAPTER ONE

Laying the Groundwork
Service and Activism

At nine o'clock on 20 December 1995, a Wednesday morning, I arrived at my office at McMaster University, Hamilton, Ontario. A fax message from Barbados awaited me from Dame Nita Barrow, with her signature R. Nita, telling me that arrangements had been made for my stay with her and that I would be met at the airport. Attached to the page was a separate piece of paper with a handwritten note from her private secretary, Pat Layne, to say that after Dame Nita had written her fax she had fallen ill and had to be hospitalized. I called Pat Layne immediately, only to be told that Dame Nita had died the night before. My fax was the last note that she had written. Pat told me that Nita's signature was perfect on this, her last message sent to me. I was overcome with emotion and wept bitterly at the news of her death. It was such a shock coming, as it did, on the heels of her message and immediately before my impending visit to Barbados to continue her oral history.

Who was Dame Nita? And why should I cry so much? After all, she was neither a family member nor a close friend. But therein lies the secret of this remarkable woman – her capacity to make every person who met her think that they were special to her. Indeed, she exuded so much warmth and caring with an unassuming demeanour that even the man who sold coconuts at the corner of her house (then the governor general's residence) would weep along with the multitude who paid their respects to her while she lay in state.

Nita Barrow, late governor general of Barbados, was born on 15 November 1916 at Nestfield, St Lucy, Barbados. The social structure of the Barbadian society into which she was born was shaped by the plantation system and slavery. More than any other West Indian island after slavery ended, Barbadian society mirrored its metropolis, Victorian England, in its class system which was modified by slavery and colour. A similar hierarchy existed in 'little England', as other West Indian territories named the island. At the top were the white plantation owners and the professionals in law, church and state; next was the middle class, a group of mixed race, the coloureds, and blacks, stratified by income; and at the bottom was the majority of the black people.[1]

Nita was the second child, and first girl, of Ruth and Reginald Barrow, in a family of five children – three girls and two boys: Graham, the eldest; Nita; Ena, who followed in Nita's footsteps and became a nurse; Errol; and Sybil, who became a pharmacist. An awareness of being first and foremost a West Indian permeated all of Nita's life. Her father was an Anglican minister whose ministry took him to many of the islands, and it happened that the children were born in three different islands – Barbados, St Vincent and the American Virgin Islands. Nita told an amusing anecdote about travelling to Europe with her second sister, Sybil, who was born in the American Virgin Islands and had an American passport. She said, "In the days when we were still colonies, if you had a British passport when you got to England you were in one line and if you had an overseas, another. We had a standing joke. She and I were travelling together and we got to this immigration officer who looked at her and said to us, 'Are you related?' and she said, 'Yes'. We did not realize why. But he said, 'One's American and the other's British.' Then he said, 'You are sisters?' And Sybil said, quick as a flash, 'Yes! Same father, same mother!' " Nita's mother's family came from Tobago and her father's family came from St Vincent. Consequently, "we say we are a West Indian family. We never grew up with the thing of being strictly Barbadian."

Nita's father was posted to St Croix, in the American Virgin Islands, where there was a growing population of West Indians who were Anglicans. Emigration had long been seen by West Indians as a major strategy for finding a better life. Her father advocated better wages for the local people and he was an outspoken critic of racism. D. Hamilton Jackson, a local patriot, was the editor/publisher of a newspaper in St Croix, the *Herald*. As editor, he wrote about the deplorable and inhuman conditions associated with the plantation system. Nita's father began to write for the newspaper and his criticisms of the inequalities in the society and the administration were published in the *Herald*. He worked with the local people to form cooperatives and buy estates for themselves. As a result of this, Revd Reginald Barrow was deported "because he was a [British] non-islander getting involved in local [American] politics". With the help of friends, he went to the United States.

The family decided then that it would be better for Ruth and the children to return to Barbados where they would get better schooling and have the support of many of the extended family of Nita's mother, the O'Neals, who were financially secure. As Nita has put it, "You know there is a tradition in those islands that there is nowhere in the Caribbean better for school than your own island, whether it is Trinidad or Barbados."

The O'Neals were comfortably well-off and also propertied. Nita's mother, Ruth, had herself attended a first-grade secondary school as a fee-paying student. This was unusual. At that time, the three fee-paying high schools for boys were the exclusive domain of the sons of the well-to-do whites who were educated in the island. Generally, the children of the upper class whites were educated in England. The coloured and the blacks or lower class, however, deemed education important for both sexes. Apart from its usefulness in their daily occupations, it was also seen as a means of increasing the respect they could earn from the white population.

Even though the black community encouraged the education of girls, racism and sexism permeated all aspects of the dominant society. Just as sons of white families received secondary education before the daughters, patriarchy gave black boys the privilege of receiving secondary education before girls were given that opportunity. Harrison College, Codrington College and the Lodge School, distinguished secondary schools for white boys, were established in 1721 and 1733 but there was no equivalent girls' school until 1881 when Queen's College was established. In the early 1900s, Nita's father was one of the few black boys who attended Codrington College, where he studied theology.[2] Higher education was limited to the few black male students who won the Barbados Scholarship and entered university at Oxford or Cambridge. The Island Scholarship system was not only competitive but profoundly antisocial. Since scholarships were few, many coloured and black middle-class families determined to send their sons to England for higher education as doctors and lawyers.[3] Nita's uncle, Duncan O'Neal, had placed second in the Barbados Island Scholarship in 1899 and was one of those whose family ensured that he had a university education. He went to Edinburgh where he studied medicine and won the gold medal in surgery.

It comes as no surprise, then, that Nita had a solid educational foundation. Her first five years of schooling, until she was ten years old, was at the dame school in

St Croix. On the family's return to Barbados, Nita attended Miss Taitt's School, which, in the tradition of those days, was a black girls' school. She was fortunate to have been born to a middle-class family. Later it would afford her the 'privilege' of being able to attend a fee-paying secondary school for black and coloured girls.

In 1923 Nathaniel Bullen, one of the first black men to be elected churchwarden of the vestry of St Michael's Cathedral, had proposed a motion to establish such a school. Since it appeared to be a revolutionary idea, it required the support of some of the liberal white lawmakers. Bullen wanted to ensure that the proposal received the support of the House of Assembly, and so a meeting of electors was called to determine their stand. The proposal met with overwhelming approval. The site chosen for the new school had once been the property of a wealthy white family and later the home of Grassfield School, a formerly exclusive all-white girls' secondary school. When St Michael's Girls' Secondary School was eventually opened in 1928, the first secondary school for black and coloured girls in Bridgetown, Miss Taitt transferred her pupils, including Nita and Ena Barrow, to the new school. These girls became the nucleus of the first group of students, and Nita proudly claimed that she and her sisters were founding members of St Michael's. Her two great-nieces would attend that school and one was still at St Michael's at the time of our planned interview. The school maintained high standards and the teachers were of very good calibre, including Miss Taitt who joined the staff and later became one of the school's outstanding headmistresses. Nita remained there for seven years, successfully completing both her junior and senior exams, set and marked by Cambridge University, following the colonial pattern. She received a Grade I Senior Cambridge School Certificate in July 1934.

Nita's sense of humour came readily to the fore when she said that Miss Taitt had told her that she was "cut out for teaching, so the minute I finished my Senior [exams], she insisted that I stay on the next term – I was not yet eighteen – and teach. Well! You know you do as you're told in those days, so I thought, great! But, my dear, I always tell her, when I had all those exercise books to correct every night and four hours of preparation to stay ahead of the students, I did not think it was funny at all!" Nita did stay on to teach for two terms and then left to begin her nursing career.

Dr Duncan O'Neal, Nita's uncle, had his office next door to the family home. Nita "would wander in and out of there but I can't tell anybody that I really was looking at being a nurse". Yet her uncle's social and political activism would have had an impact on her.

After Dr O'Neal had graduated from Edinburgh University, he had worked in Newcastle in the north of England, in Trinidad and Tobago, and in Dominica. During his studies in Scotland, he witnessed the struggles of socialism, the growth of trade unions and the progress of the Independent Labour Party, which impressed him. His practice in Newcastle was spent working among the poor and socially deprived. While in Trinidad, he became involved in community activism, working closely with Audrey Jeffers, a well-known social worker and activist for the poor and downtrodden blacks. On his return to Barbados in 1924, he became seriously involved in the workers' movement to improve the lives of the poor and underprivileged. He found that conditions had changed little in terms of working class health and sanitary facilities since his departure as a student in 1899. He was particularly disturbed by the colony's high and rising infant mortality rate and the generally poor health standards within the black communities. It was no wonder that he took up the cudgel to champion the cause of the masses.

Dr O'Neal was determined to awaken the political consciousness of the people. In 1924 he found the necessary support and interest among a number of people who were willing to rally around the new movement, which became known as the Democratic League – the first political party in Barbados. It was modelled after the British Labour Party and became the precursor of later movements. It is said to have played a considerable part in spreading the gospel of the need for adult suffrage, compulsory education, workers' compensation, and health and unemployment benefits into every parish and every village. O'Neal is credited with providing the leadership for the intellectual and political changes in Barbados in the first half of the twentieth century.

A more obvious reason for Nita's entry into nursing appears to have come from three of Nita's friends, Sybil Simmons, whose father was a doctor and a friend of Duncan O'Neal, Grace Thorne and Ivy Sealy, whose father was also a doctor. The three girls had decided to go into nursing in Barbados. Ivy Sealy's mother led a very active social life, giving lots of parties, and Nita and her friends went to many of these gatherings. Nita's main concern at that time was that "our social life was not curtailed" by going into nursing! Her friends assured her that they would still be able to get home to parties and encouraged her to apply. She was interviewed by the matron of the Barbados General Hospital and agreed to enter the programme. The fact that there had been registration for nurses in Barbados since 1932, long before the other Caribbean islands, seems to have been a favourable contributing factor. Nita had not told anyone in the family that she had decided to go into nursing. At the time, her mother was with her father in the United States, so Nita wrote to Ruth, whose advice to her was "Whatever you start, you have to finish." Before she was married, Ruth had thought of going into nursing and then work on the island of Bequia where there was a lack of doctors and nurses, but her parents would not permit her to do so. She was allowed, however, to go to the hospital in Bridgetown and observe. Nita recalled that during her training at the Barbados General Hospital, she met doctors and nurses who knew her mother from the time when she paid her visits for observation.

Dr Duncan O'Neal was on the hospital board when Nita decided to enter nursing. He knew what a difficult occupation it was, as well as the politics involved with the administration of the programme, of which Nita was totally unaware. He did not believe that Nita would stay and so he did not take her entry into the training programme seriously. The family had divided opinions on whether she was going to stay or not, but she was determined to stay, no matter how tough it was. And persist she did.

It was not unusual that Nita went into nursing, as there were few opportunities or professions open to black women then. They could get married and raise a family or go into teaching or nursing. In fact, if they married during training they were not allowed to continue. Bank jobs were occupied primarily by whites, and coloureds were being only gradually accepted. The civil service offered some technical jobs.

Less than a decade before Nita embarked on a nursing career, housing, health and sanitary conditions in Barbados were in decline with high mortality and morbidity rates, especially among the impoverished black people, and were caused mainly by epidemics of typhoid fever, yellow fever, malaria and diarrhoea. Infant mortality soared, ranging from 217 to 222 per 1,000 live births as a result of diseases such as neonatal tetanus, enteritis, congenital syphilis and prematurity. Many of these deaths were attributed to the lack of trained midwives. Births outside Bridgetown were still attended by village women who acted as midwives. Their skills had been passed on from one generation to another since the days of slavery. They lacked knowledge of aseptic techniques and the women were delivered in unhygienic conditions. Hospital conditions were just as deplorable. The black nurses worked long hours, were poorly paid, lived in atrocious dormitories, had substandard meals and functioned under outdated rules. In 1926 the Public Health Commission was appointed to examine the condition of public health in the island. The commission made sweeping recommendations for the reorganization of public health services, among them the need for training public health nurses and midwives as a means of bringing about effective improvement in public health. As usual, the recommendations were slow to be implemented.

The period between the two world wars, 1918–39, saw the rise of a number of black individuals with a social conscience and the agitation of the black masses in most of the West Indies which culminated in the riots of 1937 and 1938. It was inevitable, then, that there would be a political awakening of the nurses. The restlessness and agitation among the nurses for better working conditions, higher salaries and better standards of living was a reflection of what was happening in the society at large. Many nurses purposely broke existing rules as a sign of protest, knowing that they would be suspended; others resigned after breaking the oppressive regulations. Many senior nurses resigned to take up positions in the prison, the leprosarium, and almshouses. Yet others emigrated to the United States. Some took up private practice, caring for the sick in their homes or as private nurses for wealthy hospitalized patients. In the face of this grave situation, the colonial authorities were forced to consider the recommendations contained in the Public Health Commission's Report of 1926.[4]

The militant action of the nurses was, in fact, the catalyst for action to remedy the situation. By 1931 a sister tutor had been recruited from England to be responsible for the training of nurses and, in 1932, the Nurses and Midwives Registration Act came into being, requirinq hospitals to employ trained registered nurses. The Nursing Council was formed with responsibility for prescribing the training for nurses and midwives, discipline and registration.

The registered sister tutor (nurse educator) who had been recruited for the Barbados General Hospital was a Miss Mary Page. She arrived in Barbados in February 1932, the first trained tutor of nurses in the island, and the first to introduce formal training for the probationer nurses at the general hospital. Lectures were scheduled, classes were organized and teaching aids such as skeletons, models and anatomical charts were sent from England. Within a week of Miss Page's arrival, lectures had been organized in anatomy and physiology, hygiene, and the theory and practice of nursing. The Nursing Council used the syllabus of the General Nursing Council for England and Wales as a prototype, and a committee was formed to conduct registration examinations. There were two examinations: the preliminary examination, which was conducted after students had been in training for eighteen months; and the final examination, conducted at the completion of the programme, in effect, at the end of the third year. The examinations consisted of both theory and practical components. In the first year of operation, the papers were set by a physician, and the practical examination was conducted by two English nursing sisters (senior nurses). The novelty of the first formal programme generated much interest within the hospital, with many doctors offering to assist the sister tutor with setting and correcting examination papers and conducting the oral and practical examinations.

The administrative structure of nursing at the Barbados General Hospital, now known as the Queen Elizabeth Hospital, consisted of five key positions at the senior supervisory levels: the matron; the assistant matron; the night sister; the theatre sister; and the sister tutor, all of whom came from England. The next level consisted of Barbadian senior nurses, who were in charge of the wards. Finally, there were the staff nurses and student nurses. The hierarchical structure replicated the prevailing social and class structure of the society, with the colonial whites at the top, followed by the Barbadian whites, and then the blacks as the nurses and students at the bottom of the hierarchy.

Standards of patient care followed a similar pattern. There were two very different standards of care: one for the white upper class who had private rooms, and the other for the majority of the poor black and coloured people who occupied the bulk of the general wards of the hospital. The quality of care on the private wards was comparable to that in the private wards in England where medical and nursing care was individualized, and patients had all the amenities they would have had at home, including fine linen, silver, china and cocktails with dinner, unless contraindicated by the attending physician. The atmosphere was conducive to recovery and the patients were treated as individuals, with respect and courtesy. The general wards, by contrast, were severely overcrowded. Patients were viewed as bed numbers or objects, often nameless, and many of the basic amenities were lacking. E.K. Walters described it this way:

Admission to these wards was a traumatic experience for most people; there was an immediate loss of identity, and everywhere the atmosphere contributed to depersonalization of the people; patients were generally addressed as bed numbers, except on rare occasions when the surname was used, the accepted titles of Miss, Mrs and Mr were never used in this section of the Hospital . . . the prevailing conditions on these wards . . . caused the Hospital to be viewed by a large section of the population as a place of last resort . . .[5]

Nursing practice, then as now, was greatly influenced by the prevailing health problems. In the early 1930s, typhoid fever, tuberculosis and pneumonia were among the major diseases. Patients remained ill for long periods and many of the techniques were laborious. Shortage of supplies meant that nurses often had to improvise, and the fact that nursing staff was inadequate meant that the delivery of nursing care was not an easy task. Some of the procedures were time consuming, such as the oil meal poultice used for patients with pneumonia. Nurses had to mix, make and spread the poultice which was kept on the patient's chest by an item of clothing called the 'pneumonia jacket'. Eventually the jacket was replaced by the kaolin poultice, a premixed medicated poultice available in tins and merely requiring to be heated and spread. An epidemic of typhoid fever required that the critically ill patients who had continuous high fever and delirium be treated by the students and nurses with frequent sponge baths and ice caps to the head to bring the fever down. Continuous feeding was needed and careful observation was required of the patient's condition, especially at the critical third week when the complication of intestinal bleeding could occur. Early recognition of this could be the deciding factor between life and death. The care of patients after surgery was equally challenging, especially postoperatively. Anaesthetics at that time were chloroform and ether which caused much vomiting and restlessness. The postoperative care of patients was most demanding as they remained in bed for three weeks after abdominal surgery and, in the absence of appropriate beds, it required two or three nurses to help to position the patients comfortably. Students were petrified at the use of leeches to the eyes of patients with elevated eye tension. They had to learn to master the technique of getting the leech to bite and to maintain sucking until the prescribed time had elapsed as well as removal of the leech and its subsequent care.[6]

These were the conditions in place when Nita and the six other young women with her were admitted for training at the Barbados General Hospital. They were the first to enter as a group. Formerly, applicants had been taken in haphazardly, whenever the need arose for a pair of helping hands. The basic qualification was only a primary education and training had been, in effect, an apprenticeship. The probationers, as the nurses in training were then called, signed on for five years, although the training was supposedly for three years. They were sent to the wards from the first day and learned by doing, by trial and error, modelling, observing, and from demonstrations given by the charge nurse, depending on her whim and fancy. Learning was serendipitous. They worked a twelve-hour shift with one evening off early. However, they no longer had to wait for lectures until a group had collected or until the doctor was free.

By the time Nita's group arrived, there were regular lectures to be attended, which took them away from the wards for about two hours a week, and examinations to be passed before a nurse could be registered. Their sister tutor was a Miss Nance Purvis who had replaced Miss Mary Page. She first brought applicants in as a group and developed more structured classes. She was also instrumental, with the collaboration of the matron and the resident surgeon, in arranging refresher courses for the charge nurses and the senior nurses in the hospital. In addition, in 1938 Dr Cato, a black obstetrician from St Vincent, volunteered to give lectures in midwifery with a final examination set by him as there was no formal midwifery training in the island at the time. These lectures were most useful to the nurses as they increased their skills and knowledge in an area that was sorely needed, given the high infant and maternal morbidity that still persisted in the colony, despite the recommendations emanating from the Public Health Commission in 1926 and which were reinforced by the report of the Moyne Commission of 1938.

After the agitation and upheavals throughout the West Indies in 1937 and 1938, the Moyne Commission had been set up to investigate social and economic conditions in all the colonies and to make recommendations. The subsequent recommendations covered a sweeping range of socioeconomic concerns, including political reform. Seven of the recommendations dealt with public health and among them was the training of nurses. The implementation of many of the recommendations was delayed until after the war ended in 1945. However, improvements in the health sector in the Caribbean were seen before then, notably in public health training for nurses.

Nita remembered that probationers were sent to the wards from their first day. They usually went to the children's ward, where feeding the children and washing their cups were part of their duties. She added, "If you were fortunate to have a good charge nurse, you learned a lot; if you drew [had] one of the charge nurses who was angry at what they called 'these new-fangled ideas' because you had to leave the ward to go to a lecture at a certain time, or if you had one of the good ones as I did, a Nurse Chandler, who only just died – she was buried a month ago – she showed you everything as she talked, so you did not get this fear of being left [alone] and not knowing what to do. But if you met some of the older ones, they were angry at what they called 'these little nurses who come to take away me cap'.

You know, in those days, we were the big four and were senior and had a better basic education. Naturally, they figured we were going for interviews. Now I realize [that] for them you were a threat." The secondary education that these probationers had would present a greater threat. Secondary education, as has been pointed out earlier, had not been available for black girls and when it was introduced, few could afford to pay the fees. In the hospital, local black nurses were only just moving into charge nurse positions and those who had waited for such a long time to get there would certainly resent any perceived threat to their status.

Change is never easy for anyone. Traditionally and up to the present day, nurses as a group have real difficulty in dealing with and accepting change. Curriculum changes, the length of the nursing programmes, the location of the programmes, whether they should be hospital, college or university based have met with pockets of great resistance. This is a universal phenomenon. It was not too surprising, then, to find that the nurses who had trained in a system that allowed them no fixed time for lectures would be upset at those who seemingly had it 'easier' now that student nurses could leave the ward while on duty to attend a lecture for an hour or two.

The training course for nurses was supposed to be three years in duration, but applicants signed on as probationers for five years. The implied intent was to repay some of the cost of the training given. They were paid a stipend of sixteen shillings and sixpence a month (twenty shillings made one pound sterling). By Nita's third year, they were getting one pound a month, but the hospital withheld two shillings of that in the event that students broke a utensil. Ilene Murray Ainsley, who followed Nita in training two years later and who went on to become the first local black sister tutor in the island, was a good friend of Nita. Ilene recounted that there was a great deal of breakage of plates in the hostel. Nita had been blamed for breaking a plate, which apparently she had not, and her money was withheld. "She went to the hostel and picked up a plate and broke it and said, 'Now I've paid for it!' When you broke a bedpan, it was even worse. They were porcelain and the cost was more like twenty shillings. That was plenty of money."[7] Nita's sense of justice and fair play and courage always asserted itself in words and actions.

All the nurses and student nurses lived in residence. The juniors had a dormitory called 'Cherry Village', which they all laughed about. Then there were the middle quarters for the senior students, the married women's quarters for the most senior ones, the charge nurses, and the night dormitory where the student nurses lived when they were on night duty.

Because most of the meals were so inadequate, Nita's family often sent snacks or a full meal which would be shared with her colleagues. Nita described how her brother, Errol (who later was to become prime minister of Barbados) often came on his bicycle, bringing meals and snacks for her. Naturally, she and her friends shared the goodies. Ilene remarked that all the students used to gather at Nita's home when they were off duty. "She had a cousin, Gordon Barrow, and he used to bring some of the boys from the Air Force and we would assemble there. And Nita would always cook. She was the best cook!" This reference to Nita's flair for cooking would be repeated by many of her colleagues.

In 1937, while Nita and her group were still in training, a new nurses' residence, the Nightengale Nurses' Home, was built. The Nightengale family of Barbados, white 'Bajans', evidently no relation to Florence Nightingale, had bequeathed half of their estate to the hospital to erect a home for nurses in Barbados. The building was strongly constructed of cut and baked Barbados limestone, with a brick from the original Nightengale Home in London in the main living room.[8] With the opening of the Nightengale Home, Nita and her cohort were finally able to move to more pleasant surroundings after three years in the dormitories. The home had its own staff of cooks and maids and, as a result, meals were greatly improved.

Nita and her group found nursing hard work but because they all supported one another she never found it tedious. They all felt, however, that had they known beforehand how laborious nursing would be, they would never have entered the training programme. Nevertheless, the fact that their families did not think they would stay was a challenge and they wanted to prove that they could stay the course. There were tears of grief at night over the arduous tasks given to them on the wards and they all wanted to pack their bags and go home. The conditions of service were onerous, so that many other young women left without completing their training. Before the Nightengale Home was built, there had been housekeeping chores as well, but although the girls would come off duty tired they would shower, dress and go to whatever party was on. At that time, some of the young West Indian medical practitioners, Dr Arnot Cato from St Vincent, Dr Will Carr from Grenada and Dr Stewart, a Barbadian, had returned from their studies abroad and were assigned as juniors to the Barbados General Hospital. Nita and her friends were the 'clique' that socialized together. On duty, they pretended they did not know each other, since the rigid prevailing British system separated their professional from their personal life. Of the seven students who entered nursing with Nita only two graduated, the other five, in spite of their determination, left three months before the end of the last term. It had proved too much for them. Only

Nita and Grace Thorne graduated. It is to Nita's credit that she persisted and, as she did, with the support she received from her first ward sister, Eunice Griffith (Chandler), who encouraged her to remain. However, she intended to stay only long enough to get through as she wanted to pursue further studies.

Those who graduated in 1938 were entitled to receive their certificates in 1940. It will be recalled that the graduates had to work as payment-in-kind students for two years after their apprenticeship was over. However, the matron had the practice of withholding the certificates of the graduates after they had completed their apprenticeship. This was a major handicap to the graduates as it meant they were unable to seek employment elsewhere. This policy was yet another example of racism and classism where the white English matrons had the power over the local black nurses to withhold their certificates as they wished. With the war in progress, it was impossible to recruit senior personnel from England. At the same time, nurses could no longer go to England for postgraduate experience. This fact was apparent to the colonial leaders. Withholding their certificates was a means of retaining cheap labour for maximum work.

Early Leadership

Nita's leadership abilities were quickly recognized at Barbados General Hospital. Her assertiveness and political 'savvy' could be seen even as a student. She was not only appointed a student member of the executive of the Registered Nurses' Association, which had come into being in 1937, but was also placed in charge of the theatre. It was a very demanding position as she worked five or six nights with one additional daytime tour of duty as the 'scrub' nurse.[9]

Nita recalled that, "Finally, three or four of us, they used to call us the troublemakers, we decided it was time that we had our certificates." Since the matron had not given any of the nurses their certificates after five years in the hospital, they decided that they were going to have their own graduation. So twelve of them, from different years, who had not got their certificates planned the first graduation ever held at the Barbados General Hospital. They invited their lecturers and friends and had a party. The authorities were astounded at their assertiveness and gave them their certificates. As early as this point in young Nita's life, her sense of fairness was reminiscent of her uncle Duncan O'Neal and her father's political social activism and consciousness. After this ceremony, decisions were made by the graduates as to their future plans. Most stayed on staff but Nita was not interested in doing so. She left the Barbados General Hospital and did "a bit of private practice", but she had a thirst for knowledge and wanted more advanced training.

While Nita was in charge of the operating room theatre, she met Nora Cotton (Stoute), a graduate of the School of Nursing at the University of Toronto, the first Canadian to serve as a sister and supervisor at the hospital. This change in the leadership from the British to Canadian was a direct result of World War II. The war created a shortage of British-trained sisters, who had previously been sent out by the Colonial Office in London for senior posts at the Barbados General Hospital. Consequently, Canada as a member of the Commonwealth was the next logical choice as a source for supervisory staff. The difference in the approach of the Canadian nurses to the Barbadian nurses, compared to the British, was evident. Canadians treated Barbadian nurses as equals. Perhaps it was because Canada was also one of the colonies, although arguably racism existed within the social, economic and political life of Canada. In the course of conversation, Nita shared with Nora her dream of wanting to go abroad for further studies. It was impossible to go to Great Britain because of the war. In any case, financial assistance from the Colonial Office in London would not be available. Nora told her of the post-basic nursing programme at the University of Toronto and about the Rockefeller Foundation scholarships, based in New York, which sponsored 'good' nurses from Latin America and other parts of the world to do specified post-basic nursing courses.

The University of Toronto was, at that time, one of the few universities in North America that was both innovative and flexible with regard to nursing education. The School of Nursing had designed post-basic programmes for graduate nurses to prepare them for leadership positions in public health, nursing administration and nursing education. These programmes were unique in that certificates from other nursing jurisdictions outside Canada were considered to be a valid qualification for entry into the Toronto School of Nursing. The course in public health nursing was particularly renowned as it had its early beginnings as a subdepartment in the School of Hygiene. This arrangement provided a distinct advantage for the Department of Public Health Nursing as it provided an association with a strong programme of research and teaching in a school that had gained wide recognition and respect for its contribution to preventive medicine and public health. The Rockefeller Foundation had financially supported and encouraged the School of Nursing since the early 1930s. The president of the foundation considered Toronto to be one of the top schools for nursing training in the world.[10] Dr Kathleen Russell's (director of the School of Nursing) leadership, scholarly ability and insight into the nursing needs of the community had produced an outstanding research programme. Moreover, the foundation was supportive of providing scholarships for nurses internationally to attend the preventive medicine and public health programme at the University of Toronto because of its outstanding reputation. Selection of the nurses sponsored was based upon their potential for ultimately holding leadership positions in institutions in their country of origin.

Nita acted promptly on Nora's suggestion and wrote to her mother in New York. Her uncle 'Ebie', Ebenezer O'Neal (her mother's brother), who also lived in New York, made enquiries for her and took her letter of application to the Rockefeller Foundation.

Meanwhile, Nita had heard of an excellent formal course in midwifery in Trinidad conducted by Dr Waterman. Dr Cato in Barbados had introduced lectures in midwifery during her time in the programme there, but his was not a formally recognized course. In addition, only the abnormal cases went to the Barbados General Hospital, while the normal deliveries went to the almshouse where students were sent for their practical experience. Nita made up her mind to go to Trinidad to take the midwifery course there. The Barbados Registered Nurses' Association, through its president Eunice Gibson, had made arrangements for the colonial hospital in Trinidad to assist in training some of its members in midwifery. In 1940 Nita set out for Trinidad for her midwifery training. On her return to Barbados after the successful completion of the programme, she received a reply from the Rockefeller Foundation requesting her to go to Trinidad to be interviewed by one of their staff, Dr Dowens, head of the epidemiological unit, on behalf of the Rockefeller Foundation. So she had to make another trip to Trinidad.

At that time there were no interisland flights in the Caribbean. Travel between the islands was by boat, a rough adventure, to say the least. Cramped quarters on these boats for a day and a half with the wind, sea spray and possibly seasickness did not promise a pleasurable experience. Fortunately, there were the 'Lady' boats – *Lady Drake*, *Lady Nelson* and *Lady Rodney*. These were the ships of the Canadian

National Steamship Company which sailed between Canada and the West Indies. They had cabins available for those passengers who were willing and able to pay the price for some comfort and privacy. They carried salted codfish, lumber and assorted cargo from Canada to the various West Indian islands. On their return trip, they would carry rum, sugar and other products to Canada. Most of the local people travelled on deck where, in close proximity with one another, they shared food, drinks and blankets, and a camaraderie evolved amidst the night's chill and the sea's turbulence. The voyage on the 'Lady' boats was shorter and took about a day. It was on one of these vessels that Nita travelled to return to Trinidad for her interview. She was offered a one-year scholarship to the University of Toronto.

Her journey to Toronto in 1943, during the war years, was informative and showed her courage, confidence and willingness to take risks. After taking a 'Lady' boat to Trinidad, she had to fly via Haiti and to Miami for her connection to New York to be briefed by the Rockefeller Foundation. Servicemen, soldiers, sailors and airmen had priority on all flights and "you took your chance all alone". She was bumped off her flight and had to stop over in Haiti for two days, and when she arrived in Miami her connection to New York had long gone. She was again forced to remain a further two days there, as "you are at the will of the army, when they have any space". Miami in the 1940s was a hotbed of racism and Nita had to find accommodation. The two hotels that catered to blacks were not suitable for her. Fortunately, her friends in Trinidad had given her the name and address of a family in Miami. Nita persuaded them to accommodate her in their guest room. Her experience in Miami was one of racism such as she never encountered in Barbados. While she had somewhere to sleep, no meals were provided. She told the tale of getting on a bus after leaving a restaurant that served blacks, handing over her fare, and sitting in the front of the bus just as she normally would have done at home. The driver did not move the bus and said, "Go to the back of the bus." He repeated it a number of times but Nita did not realize that he meant her. At last he approached her and told her that he could not move the bus until she went to the back. She was not to be intimidated and boldly responded that the back of the bus was full. The driver then handed her back her fare and she refused it, saying sharply, "You can keep it", and proudly got off the bus, although she was hurting inside. It was indeed ironic that almost forty or more years later, in 1986, Nita would be invited to the same city, Miami, to attend an American Jewish Committee meeting and to receive an award in recognition of her contribution to peace and her special skills as convenor of the United Nations Decade of Women Conference in Nairobi the previous year.

She finally arrived in New York, four days late, to find her uncle frantic. She stayed one week there with her aunt, Hugh Springer's mother,[11] before going on to the University of Toronto to take the one-year post-basic course in public health nursing.

Public health was clearly a long-standing need in the Caribbean. That first year there were ten students in the programme, including international students from Latin America, Australia, and India, but Nita was the only one from the Caribbean. There were, however, West Indian students in other disciplines at the university who greeted her warmly. Among them was Eugenia Charles who had arrived in 1942 and was pursuing the four-year bachelor's degree programme before completing her studies in law at the Inns of Court in London. In later years she would become Dame Eugenia and prime minister of Dominica. Ivy Baxter was there also, studying physical education through the sponsorship of the Young Women's Christian Association (YWCA), and also Ivy Lawrence (Maynier).

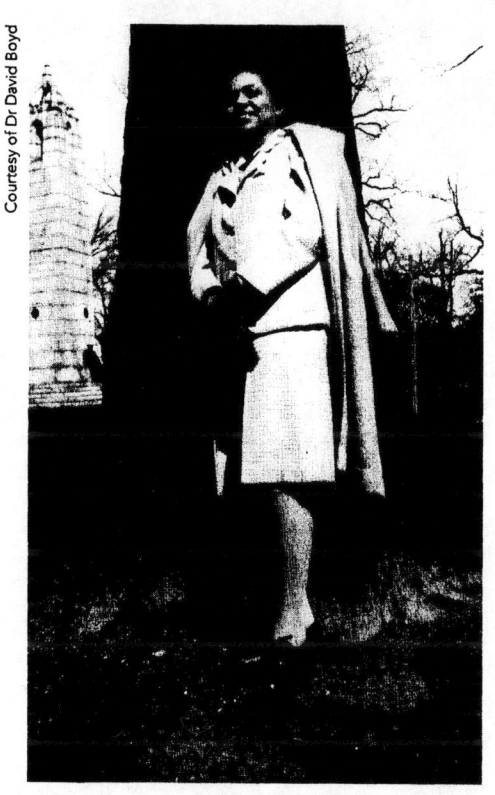

Nita Barrow on the grounds of University of Toronto, April 1944

Several young West Indian men were also students at that time. They included David Boyd from St Kitts who was studying dentistry. His recollections of those days and of Nita were that "she was a live wire when it came to having fun . . . after the day was done. She might have been doing nursing but it seemed to me that she had a lot to do with the culinary aspect because the two (Nita and Eugenia Charles) agreed to put on a West Indian feast and I personally loved it because the Canadian fare was not quite my, shall I say, cup of tea."[12]

19

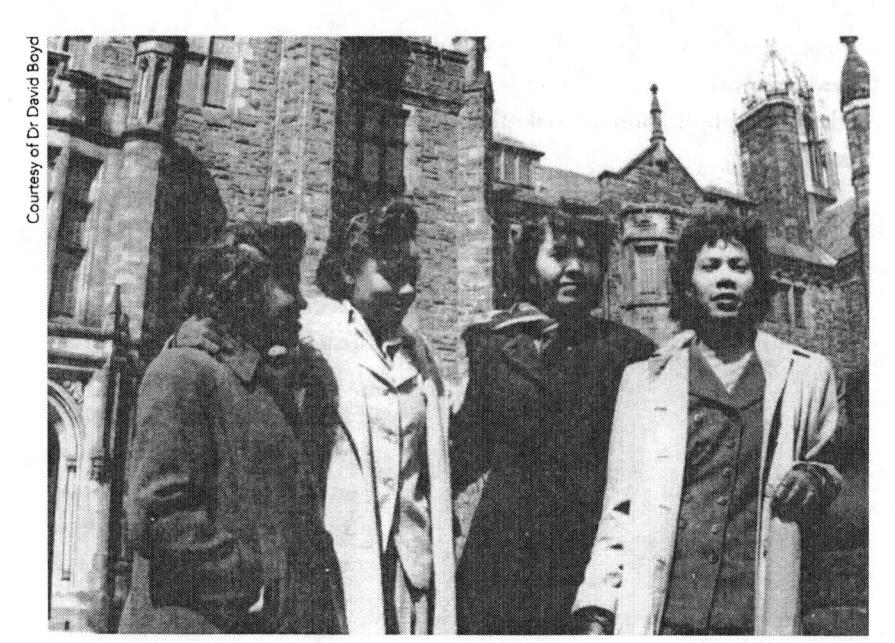

Nita and friends, University College, University of Toronto, April 1944. From left to right: Ivy Lawrence, Nita Barrow, Wilma Cameron, Eugenia Charles

The West Indian students, male and female, were a small and tightly knit group who met regularly for parties and outings together. A real camaraderie developed between them. The experience of the long cold winters and the fact that they were a visible minority from the West Indies created a bond between them. Some of the West Indian families who lived permanently in Toronto opened their homes to them for gatherings of one kind or another and this helped to make their student days enjoyable.

Nita had expected to return to the Caribbean on completion of her year of study. However, she was invited to be the valedictorian at the graduation dinner. She chose to speak on the training of nurses in Barbados and the state of public health in the island. During the function, she was approached by Miss Tennant, an advisor with the Rockefeller Foundation. Miss Tennant had been very impressed with Nita's presentation and was aware of the fact that the Public Health School in Jamaica had positions available but could not find qualified West Indians to take them. She thought that Nita would be a most suitable candidate and asked her if she would stay on at the University of Toronto for a second year and focus on nursing education with teaching preparation as a main thrust. A further

Laying the Groundwork: Service and Activism

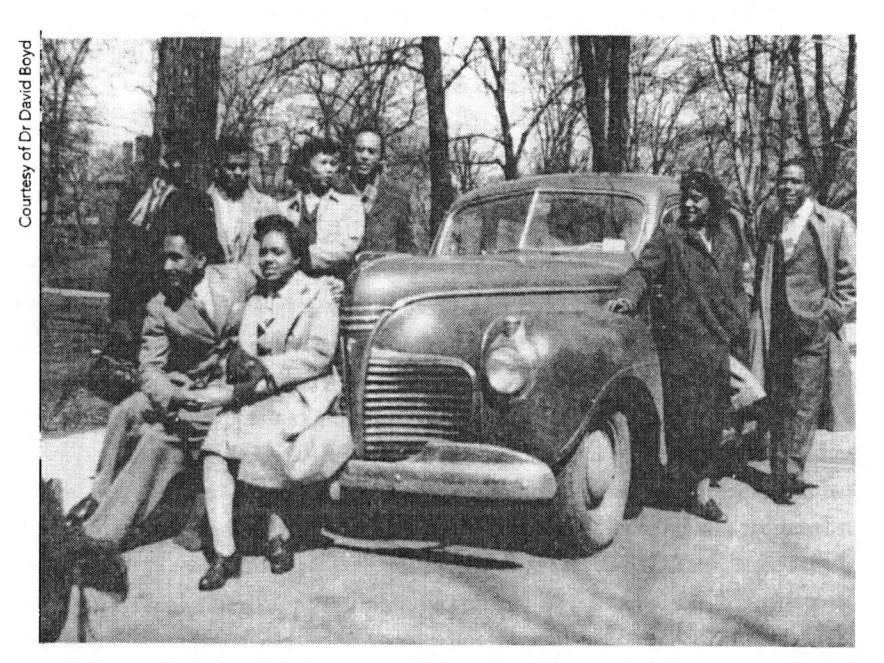

Nita and her friends, University of Toronto, 1944

scholarship from the Rockefeller Foundation made it possible for Nita to take up the offer.

A year later, in May 1945 having completed her nursing education studies, Nita was sent to Jamaica for one month of field experience and to observe public health training there, since that was where she would be working after her Canadian studies. This was a standard requirement by the Rockefeller Foundation for their scholarship students. Funding came from the foundation. Because of the lack of suitably qualified West Indian personnel, Mary Thomas, a Canadian nurse, had been sent to assist with the Jamaican public health programme.

This was Nita's first visit to Jamaica and she found the conditions on the outskirts of Kingston and in the rural areas more depressing than any she had encountered in Barbados or Trinidad. However, it provided a valuable learning experience. At the end of her month in Jamaica, Nita decided to return to Barbados for a well-earned three-month vacation. However, World War II had ended while she was there, in August, so "I took myself to Trinidad to have a real ball on VJ day." While she was there a cable arrived from the Rockefeller Foundation, offering her the position of assistant instructress with the School of Public Health in

Jamaica. Nita was not sure if that was really the job that she wanted but "it was *the* job so you took it", and agreed to stay for two years.

NITA'S JAMAICAN SOJOURN

On her arrival in Jamaica, Nita met more than she had bargained for. Mary Thomas, the Canadian nurse who had been in charge of the programme was now Mary Wolfe since, in the interim, she had married a commissioned officer in the British regiment stationed in Jamaica. Nita's arrival in the afternoon coincided with the departure of Mary and her husband for England in the morning. They had not expected to leave so soon after the war ended but the regiment had been ordered back to England. Nita said, "I arrived green to a desk as clean as the top of that table", pointing to one in her room. So here was Nita, a young, relatively inexperienced nurse, faced with heading a public health programme that she had never taught, with her sole support and advisor gone! However, she rose to the occasion. With the able assistance of two of her male colleagues at the School of Public Health, Nita got the programme under way.

Her Barbadian accent was a shock to the Jamaican nurses. More than that, there were many words that each island used or pronounced differently and that also created quite a stir when she was teaching. However, they soon learned to understand her accent and the different terminology used in Barbados and Jamaica for the same fruit or vegetable. But what was more important was that they grew to love and respect her as all who ever encountered her invariably did. Ilene Murray Ainsley was one of the students in that public health programme. Ilene said fondly, "I did my public health there. She taught me. I remember we had a child who was very sick. She was Barbadian and everyone was scared for this child but not Nita. Nita brought her from the hospital, put her in the tub, let her have a bath, and everybody was scared. But not Nita. She was that sort of person."

There were seven senior nurses who had been practising public health in Jamaica although they did not have any training. These nurses were the first to be trained, followed by nurses from other islands where public health programmes were to be developed. One of the first students in the programme told Nita a story years later. It always made Nita laugh and she chuckled while she shared it with me: "The morning that you walked in the class, we said, 'But wait! Where this little gal come from? What teacher? You think she know(s) anything?' " This has

Laying the Groundwork: Service and Activism

to be understood within the context of the island's insularity. In 1945 Jamaican nurses had little or no encounter with nurses from other islands. Nita asserted that they did not know any Barbadians in those days and that no one in the 1990s could be aware of this. Colonialism had created artificial barriers by decreeing that the avenues of communication should be between the various islands and London rather than among the territories themselves. It was once said that "a Jamaican sees more of his brethren of the other islands in six months spent in London and on shipboard between Barbados and Southampton, than in six years in his own island".[13] That was largely true up to the 1960s and helped to explain the notorious psychological alienation of Jamaicans from the eastern Caribbean islands. This was clearly a matter of communications, not geography, where the British policy of keeping the colonies apart from each other for three hundred years failed to build up a sense of West Indian nationhood. Fortunately, while certainly not perfect, in the late 1940s the University College Hospital of the West Indies (UCHWI) was a catalyst in breaking down those barriers. Subsequently, with the independence of the various territories and their determination to create Caribbean initiatives, interisland communication has improved in the 1990s.

Nita's experience in the public health programme laid the foundation for her long outstanding international career in the field of public health. It will be recalled that she had not wanted to teach, but she did teach nursing for more than ten years. She remained with the School of Public Health for five years, planning the courses and teaching some of them. The West Indies School of Public Health, opened at the Kingston Public Hospital in 1945, was designed to prepare nurses and health inspectors for the Caribbean. It had been set up as a result of the recommendations emanating from the Moyne Commission of 1938.[14]

Nita organized both the theory and the practice components of the one-year public health post-diploma nursing programme in the West Indies School of Public Health. Together with colleagues in the school, she organized the practice field: "We had to set up a programme so we could be sure . . . we had control teaching that was all put into the field with people in there. It was quite a big programme when I look at it now." One parish was selected to be used as a model unit for the field practice component of the programme. Health centres were set up, with clinics and qualified nurses in charge, and health inspectors. The students were assigned a given number of hours together and then Nita would go around and supervise them individually as well. They were taught the theory in the classroom.

During her stay at the School of Public Health, Nita observed that the nurses from Jamaica and the other Caribbean islands coming for post-basic training in public health had many learning deficiencies. They did not have a sound basis in anatomy and physiology or physics, so she was always having to patch up the gaps. In order to remedy this situation, it would be necessary to get the students into the nursing school's programmes. Knowing that there was no uniform training in the islands and that few, if any, had registration for nurses, Nita began to focus on the need for better standards in nursing education in the Caribbean. The University College of the West Indies (UCWI, later the University of the West Indies [UWI]) had come into being and was starting a medical school, "so you needed a certain standard of care". This need fitted in quite well with Nita's ideas for nursing education.

In 1945 the West Indian Committee of the Commission on Higher Education in the Colonies had recommended the establishment of a university in the British West Indies. Jamaica was chosen as the first site for that university. This was seen to be logical as Jamaica, through its pioneer welfare cooperative, Jamaica Welfare Limited, had already developed an extensive programme of adult education in the rural districts. A regional university would enable scholars to study in the Caribbean instead of British universities where the training was exemplary but largely irrelevant to West Indian needs. A medical school was a foregone conclusion as among the first faculties, so that West Indian physicians could be prepared to address the health needs of the region, since royal commission reports had repeatedly expressed concern about the state of health in the Caribbean colonies.

In fact, several health initiatives were going on simultaneously in the region during the years that the university was proposed and after it opened in 1948 as a result of the report. The School of Public Health was undergoing change in its training; the UCHWI was being constructed and opened its doors in 1952; and at about the same time seven Jamaican nurses who had gone abroad for training, during the war years, returned to the island. Two of them were appointed as assistant instructresses in the School of Public Health with Nita. Others were made sisters at the UCHWI. Only two English matrons remained in the island and they identified strongly with the Jamaican nurses.

Laying the Groundwork: Service and Activism

COLLECTIVE ACTIVISM

Once she had seen the need for better nursing education in the Caribbean, Nita realized that united action would be necessary to bring it about. Gathering a group of nurses of kindred spirit, she worked with them to form a nurses' association. It was the nucleus of what would later become the Nurses' Association of Jamaica (NAJ). For three years they met in her living room every month. Their whole filing system was held in a suitcase kept under Nita's bed. In the West Indian culture where West Indians, by and large, do not seem to hold on to things of the past, where records are destroyed, misplaced or lost, it is most heartwarming to know that the nurses of Jamaica have held on to that suitcase. It tells a story of struggle and achievement, unity and diversity; the struggle to get the NAJ off the ground; the sense of achievement in introducing registration for nurses; unity between islanders, Barbadian and Jamaican; and diversity in its formation with representation from black and white, English and West Indian. That now old brown weather-beaten, leather suitcase is a symbol of pride and joy to Jamaican nurses. It is today housed as a treasure in the headquarters of the NAJ, in the Mary Seacole Annex in Kingston. Attached to the suitcase is an inquiring label: "Can you see

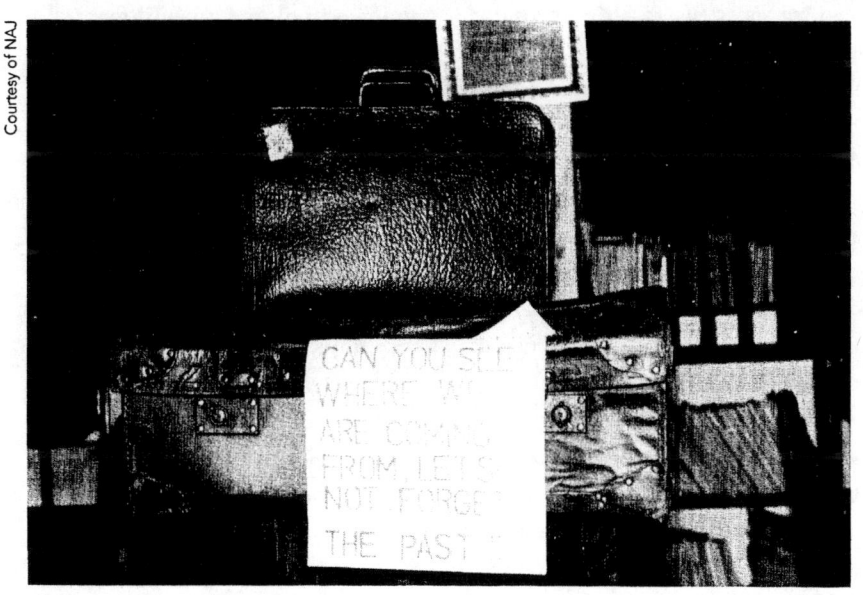

The battered, weather-beaten suitcase that Nita used to store files during the early days in the formation of the Nurses' Association of Jamaica, 1945

where we are coming from? Let's not forget the past!" A haunting reminder to nurses of the early beginnings and struggles of their nursing association.

On Friday 19 July 1946, the Jamaica General Trained Nurses' Association (JGTNA), now the NAJ, was launched with much pride, great exuberance and a spirit of commitment by all nurses. Like their counterparts in Barbados and Trinidad and Tobago, who had formed their professional nurses' associations earlier, there was the desire to gain recognition abroad, particularly from Great Britain, which was held to be the gold standard. Such recognition would be seen as an acceptance of local standards. There was a great desire among the rank and file nurses for Jamaican leaders to emerge who would promote their individual interests and encourage their belief that, given the opportunity, Jamaicans could attain great heights. Their major goals were to obtain registration for local nurses and to advance the status of nursing in Jamaica. To that end, the newly formed nurses' association requested, through the director of medical services, that representatives of the JGTNA meet formally with the two Colonial Office representatives, Blanche Shenton and Emily MacManus, who had been sent to examine standards of nursing in the colonies. At the meeting, which was attended by a delegation of Jamaican nurses headed by Nita Barrow as the president of the JGTNA, several items were on the agenda. These included educational standards for nurses, standards for training, the need for sister tutors and a preliminary training school, the establishment of an examining board with nursing representation, registration for nurses and midwifery training.

Securing registration was no easy task. Apparently, there was no pressing desire on the part of government to change the status quo, as it was to their economic advantage to continue staffing the hospitals primarily with student nurses as cheap labour. Paternalism and gender, class and racial barriers persisted. The society was paternalistic and since most physicians were men, little attention was paid to any ideas generated by nurses, almost all of whom were women. Local nurses continued to be exploited financially. Although nurses were employed by the government in the hospitals, they were not considered to be civil servants so they were denied the benefits offered to civil service employees. There was a vast difference in salaries paid to the British matrons who were sent by the Colonial Office compared to those of the local matrons. Local nurses and matrons were underpaid and had little or no status. The nurses were aware of these discriminatory practices and were determined to address these injustices so they supported the bill for registration wholeheartedly.

We see here the early beginning of feminism in nursing, where Jamaican nurses became a force to be reckoned with. The JGTNA gained recognition in the island through its clear articulation of stands on issues. Registration for nurses would result in increased credibility and status for nurses and present a challenge to the government in terms of salary demands. It would also ensure competent practitioners through improved standards of training, leading to improved health services. This realization engendered support from some within the medical profession. There was relentless lobbying on the part of the nursing leaders who showed determination and persistence as well as political savvy. There were endless negotiations and a female physician, Dr Hyacinth Lightbourne, is credited with lending both power and gender to the nurses' cause by giving it her support. Dr Lightbourne mobilized influential support for the passage of the bill through contact with Lady Foot, the wife of the governor. An audience with Lady Foot was scheduled and she received a deputation of nurses made up of some of the activists spearheading this movement. Lady Foot's interest and her support of registration for nurses were clearly seen in her offer to provide assistance in whatever way she could to facilitate passage of the bill.[15]

Nita's leadership style in words and action throughout all these endeavours was participatory and group oriented. She put it aptly: "You don't want to end up and say, I have done so and so. To me, you have to do it with a group and through a group." There was active lobbying to get the nurses' registration bill passed. There were about a dozen people working behind the scenes, nurses and some of their very good friends who were doctors would give support and share ideas with the nurses, all lobbying to get the bill passed. In August 1951 the nurses heard that the bill was going to be debated in the House and that many of the members opposed it, so they organized a representative group of nurses who were to be present in the House of Representatives during the debate. Nita was in England at the time, completing her tutor's course. When the bill was presented to the floor of the House, there was much stonewalling. Alexander Bustamante, the prime minister at that time, looked around the House and saw all the nurses in their flowing falls,[16] sitting in the visitors' gallery and looking adamant. He sent a note to Donald Sangster, who was leading the debate, saying, "Man, stop playing the fool – don't you see the women there in the gallery – they mean business!" The bill was passed that day, 15 August 1951. Such political activism on the part of the nurses led Nita to comment that "they would be called feminists now." Indeed, like black women who have historically been agents of change in their own world, the nurses played a significant role in shaping their immediate environment. Their struggle reminds us of all women's struggle against oppression and subordination, and black women in particular.

Despite the banding together of women, it took five years from 1946 for the registration bill to become law. The government feared a loss of control over nurses, which was apparent as the bill would provide for the Nursing Council to have authority for the education of nurses and give nurses more autonomy. The law eventually came into effect on 15 December 1951. It was greeted far and wide with congratulations from both lay and professional supporters. The Nursing Council for Jamaica held its first meeting on 14 January 1952, creating a new era in the history of nursing in Jamaica.

Once the JGTNA had come into being, it needed a permanent base. Land was obtained through elite contacts such as Lady Foot. She was the president of the YWCA and Nita was on the board of the YWCA, so they knew each other. Lady Foot assisted in the search behind the scenes, as did members of the Red Cross, the YWCA and the Women's Federation. Carmen Lusan, a friend of Nita's, was the general secretary of the YWCA in Jamaica and was another important contact. Finally, a site was found for the JGTNA on the same Crown land where these organizations were housed. The usefulness of having elite contacts to help achieve one's goals is exemplified here. Once the nurses were granted part of the Crown lands they had identified (on South Camp Road), a 'peppercorn' rental for ninety-nine years was arranged, and the JGTNA built their headquarters next to the Red Cross, the Women's Federation, and the YWCA. That area became the headquarters of all those primarily women's organizations. It took about three years for the land and building to materialize.

Just as Florence Nightingale used important political contacts to achieve her goals, so did Nita. Florence Nightingale would not have been able to achieve success in Crimea without powerful male political connections. However, in Nita's case she connected with women in powerful positions. This in no way implied that Nita was averse to gaining the active support of men in power positions. As she so well observed, "Life is political. Anything you want you have to work on it." This was further seen in two critical areas in the history of nursing in Jamaica and the Caribbean – the registration of nurses and the position of a principal nursing officer. The support of influential people, both men and women, was crucial for success.

Nita became the first president of this newly proclaimed JGTNA in 1946. She had a tenure of three years as president of the association, a major feat considering that she was not Jamaican. But by then, arguably, she could be considered an

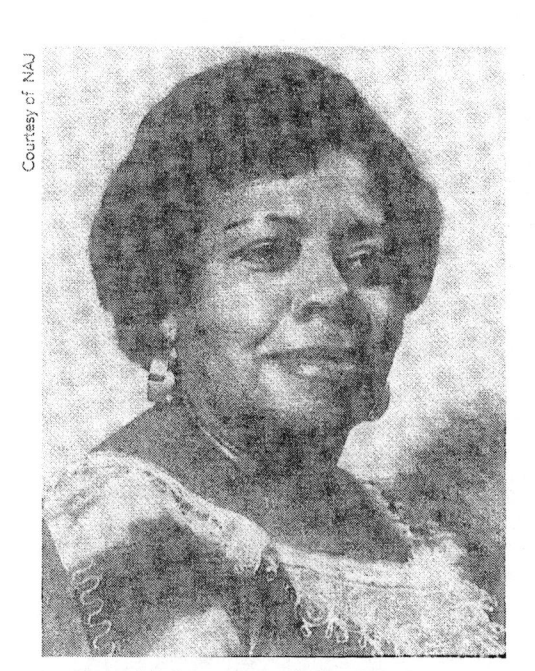

President of the Nurses' Association of Jamaica, 1946–1948

honorary Jamaican. The registration of nurses did a lot for nursing. It raised the profile of the profession, and so encouraged nurses from other islands to come to Jamaica for public health training. Nita, always modest, was adamant that these were not her achievements but the achievement of all Jamaican nurses: "I am always amused. You do not do it all alone . . . You have people who you propose the ideas to [like] doctors. I said, 'You have a strong medical association, why don't we have a nurses' association?' They said, 'Why don't you do something about it?' So you do something about it. I collected twelve like spirits . . . We had a lot of rejections . . . Even nurses don't see what we want . . . and then you get an association."

Nita noted that these accomplishments were not only Jamaican but also West Indian. Jamaica became the hub for nursing, medical and public health activities, with nurses, doctors and health inspectors from the Caribbean islands going there for studies or to teach at the School of Public Health or UWI. Many others contributed their knowledge and skills to the hospitals and the university. That era of the late forties and fifties was one of optimism and high hopes for the West Indies.

Those decades saw a number of important developments in the growth of the West Indies, politically and intellectually. It was the first time in its history that unity was seen between the islands. In a series of conferences between 1944 and 1958 the concept of political federation was brought to fruition. Unfortunately, the Federation lasted for only four years, from 1958 to 1962. When it collapsed, the West Indian territories embarked upon the task of building free nations out of British colonies. Political independence in later years created the states in which Caribbean nationhood could develop, and economic necessities forced some common action.

BREAKING THE GLASS CEILING

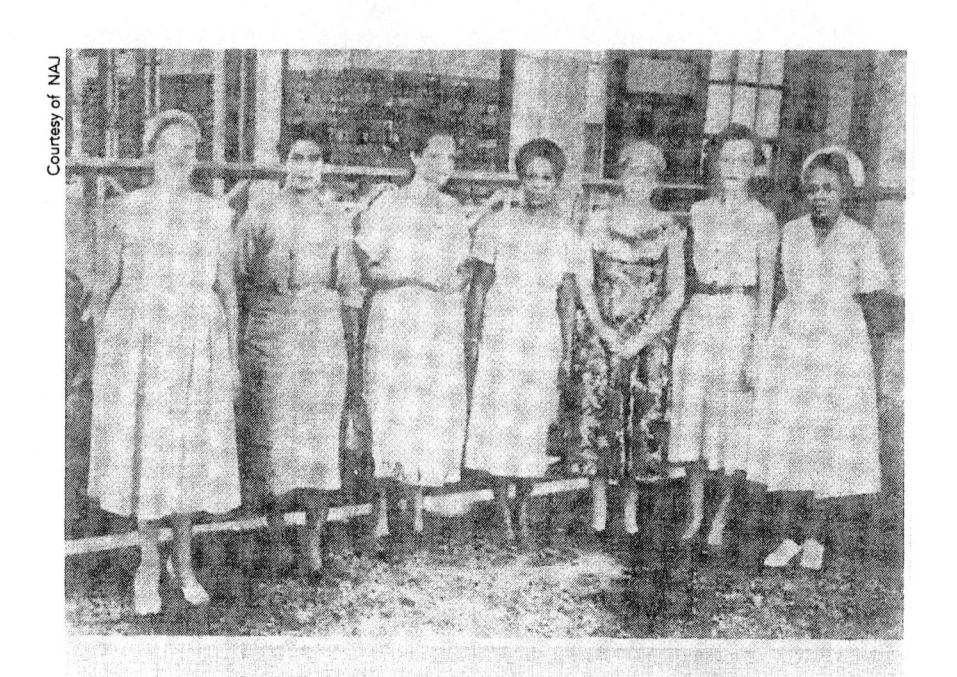

PRESIDENTS OF THE JAMAICA GENERAL TRAINED NURSES' ASSOCIATION

1946	—	MISS NITA BARROW	1951	—	MISS J. SYMES
1947	—	MISS NITA BARROW	1952	—	MISS E. LOWE
1948	—	MISS NITA BARROW	1953	—	MISS CYNTHIA VERNON
1949	—	MRS. GRACE MARCH	1954	—	MRS. VIOLET SKEFFREY
1950	—	MRS. GRACE MARCH	1955	—	MISS ZOE BURROWES
		1956	—	MRS. GRACE MARCH	

Presidents of the Nurses' Association of Jamaica, 1946–1956

Envisioning a New Dawn

In 1950 Nita was offered a Commonwealth Development and Welfare Fellowship at Edinburgh University to do a sister tutor's course. She left for a year of study at Edinburgh, arranged through the Royal College of Nursing, Edinburgh. The Royal College of Nursing, London, also offered a one-year postgraduate course for nurses to train as ward sisters, under the Colonial Development and Welfare Scheme. The main purpose of this was to prepare nurses for positions as nursing sisters for the UCHWI. It is interesting to note that this policy of offering fellowships was ultimately derived from the report of the Moyne Commission in 1938. The first result had been the appointment of a comptroller for development and welfare for the West Indies. The comptroller established the organization's headquarters in Barbados in 1940 and brought with him a staff of economic and educational experts. These experts travelled around the region, assessing the various requests for financial grants and recommending selected appropriations from the imperial treasury's Colonial Development and Welfare Fund. Public works programmes, school buildings, reservoirs, medical centres and adult education projects all received substantial help. These changes during the war years were brought about not only by the goodness of the imperial powers but also by sheer necessity. The improvements were, in part, due to real interest and concern arising out of the disclosures of the Royal Commission and, in part, in response to the criticism by the United States of Britain's treatment of her dependent empire. European imperialism was now in the shadow of American military power and was no doubt tempered by these considerations.[17] Medical and health services, of necessity, figured prominently among the schemes. These fellowships Nita and others received were supported by the imperial treasury's fund to prepare Caribbean nurses as ward sisters or sister tutors while plans were made and became realities for new teaching hospitals based upon local knowledge and the expert views of the General Nursing Council and the Royal College of Nursing.

It will be recalled that Nita had long been concerned with the deficiencies in the students' preparation when they entered the post-basic courses in public health. Remembering the words of a tutor who always said to her, "All right Nita don't complain – go do something about it", she did. She took the tutor's course, and on her return in 1951, Nita joined a team of teachers at the School of Nursing at the Kingston Public Hospital who were working to prepare students to be efficient nursing staff for the proposed UCHWI. The reorganized Kingston Public Hospital school was just beginning with a team consisting of two English tutors hired to assist Gertrude Swaby, a white Jamaican nurse who had completed post-basic nursing education at Columbia University. Their task was to organize the basic nursing education programme, which was still very inefficient, and rationalize the experiences in preparation for the three-year programme recommended by the General Nursing Council. Nita and the other tutors knew that it was imperative to improve the quality of nursing education as there was the strong possibility of a new teaching hospital – UCHWI. Nita worked for three years, until 1954, in the basic programme, getting it reorganized with Gertrude Swaby and the other team members. Nita credited Gertrude Swaby with working diligently in nursing education to improve standards in nursing. She was born in Albert Town, Trelawny, in 1912, the fourth daughter of an Anglican minister, and died in 1989. Her untiring efforts to make nursing a respected profession through sound education have been described by Syringa Marshall-Burnett as the hallmark of this woman's career.[18]

When the UCHWI opened, a number of West Indian nurses who had gone to England for preparation as ward sisters came back to work at the hospital. Some, after completion of their nursing programmes in their own respective islands, went for a year or two of additional studies. This prepared them for English registration as state registered nurses, then they chose a speciality, such as paediatrics or orthopaedics. These nurses formed a nucleus of West Indian ward sisters who helped to open the UCHWI. This was a major achievement for Caribbean nursing. At last, West Indians were having their own people in control of nursing services. A transfer of power was gradually taking place.

NOTES

1. G. Lewis, *The Growth of the Modern West Indies* (New York: Monthly Review Press, 1968), 229.
2. F.W. Blackman, *Dame Nita: Caribbean Woman, World Citizen* (Kingston, Jamaica: Ian Randle Publishers, 1995), 8.
3. Lewis, *The Growth of the Modern West Indies*, 69–94, 229.
4. H. Beckles, *A History of Barbados: From Amerindian Settlement to Nation-State* (Cambridge: Cambridge University Press, 1990), 151–60; E.K. Walters, *Nursing: A History*

from the Late Eighteenth–Late Twentieth Century Barbados (Bridgetown, Barbados: E.K. Walters, 1995), 8–12; *Report of the Committee on the Training of Nurses for the Colonies*, Cmd. 6672 (1945); *West India Royal Commission Report*, Cmd. 6607 (June 1945).

5. Walters, *Nursing: A History*, 43.
6. Ibid., 13–14.
7. Ilene Murray Ainsley, personal interview, January 1996. All material quoted from Ainsley is from this interview.
8. The Nightengale Nurses' Home later fell into some disrepair after nurses no longer lived in residences, but it has since been renovated for the use of medical students doing their residencies.
9. The scrub nurse was the nurse who assisted the surgeon in the operating room, handing the surgeon the instruments and ligatures for the surgical procedure. She had to scrub or wash her arms and hands thoroughly to ensure that they were germ-free and then put on sterile gloves.
10. H.M. Carpenter, "The University of Toronto School of Nursing: Agent of Change", in *Nursing in a Changing Society*, edited by Mary Innis (Toronto: University of Toronto Press, 1970), 94.
11. Hugh Springer, Nita's first cousin, preceded her as governor general of Barbados.
12. David Boyd, personal interview, December 1995. All material quoted from Boyd is from this interview.
13. Frank Cundall, "Jamaica" in *British America* (London: Kegan Paul, Trench, Trubner and Co., 1900), cited by Lewis, *The Growth of the Modern West Indies*, 18.
14. *West India Royal Commission Report*.
15. See P. Hay Ho Sang, "The Development of Nursing Education in Jamaica, West Indies: 1900–1975" (DEd diss., Teachers' College, Columbia University, 1984), 152–85, where the issue of registration is fully explored.
16. The fall is a traditional flowing headdress once worn by nurses, also called a veil.
17. P. Blanshard, *Democracy and Empire in the Caribbean* (New York: Macmillan), 323–26.
18. See *Jamaican Nurse* 28 (1990) where the entire issue of the journal is devoted to tributes to Gertrude Swaby for her contributions to her profession in her country.

Chapter Two

Reaching the Pinnacle

Called to the Helm

Transfer of power from the hands of the British to those of West Indians was a long-standing dream in almost all the Caribbean colonies. But when the new and long-awaited UCHWI opened in 1951, it was still a British nurse, Miss Foster Smith, who was appointed matron. When she resigned in 1954, Nita was appointed to be the first West Indian matron of UCHWI, a teaching hospital for medical students. This was a cause for much celebration not only in Jamaica but throughout the West Indies, as it was the first time in the history of the region that a local black woman was heading one of its major health institutions. At long last, West Indians were coming into their own. As matron, Nita was also responsible for the new three-year nursing programme.

Ann Jacobs, formerly matron of St Vincent Hospital, now retired and living in St Kitts, reminisced about the time that she first met Dame Nita, and the impact it had on her and her future goals. Ann and Evelyn Francis (now Lady Standard) were en route to England via Jamaica for further studies, when Nita kindly sent someone to meet them on the ship to take them ashore and go sightseeing. Ann recalled: "I was so impressed to see this young girl, Nita, lecturing to doctors, nurses, you know . . . And she was so down-to-earth, a natural person. No airs or anything. So I decided, oh my dear! I would like to be a nurse like Nita, you know. So when I got to England I kept writing to her . . . and when I heard that she was made matron of the University Hospital, I was so pleased because Miss Smith was the British matron. I was so proud: imagine that this black girl is now matron!"[1]

Ann returned to the Caribbean after her studies and indeed was inspired by Nita. Many years later she herself became the first black matron of St Vincent Hospital. She and Nita maintained their ties through the years. But Nita was not destined to stay long in the position of matron of UCHWI, prestigious as it was. A greater challenge awaited her.

At that time the organizational structure in the Ministry of Health consisted of three medical doctors – a chief medical officer and two principal medical officers. One of the principal medical officers was responsible for nursing affairs and the other was in charge of medicine. After registration had been achieved for nurses and the Nursing Council was created, which was responsible for setting the standards of theory and practice in nursing as well as conducting the registration examinations, nurses began agitating for a principal nursing officer to head nursing affairs in the island instead of a physician, the principal medical officer.

After much lobbying, the position of principal nursing officer was eventually approved and advertised. The chief nursing officer in Britain, Florence Udell, came to Jamaica to do the recruiting. In the 1950s, the British still assumed responsibility for the selection of nursing and medical personnel to fill senior administrative positions. Miss Udell approached Nita and asked her why she had not applied for the position. Nita informed her that she had only been two and a half years as matron at UCHWI and that she was enjoying it. She was taken aback to find that her name had not only been submitted but that she had, in fact, been appointed to the position. So in 1956 Nita achieved another first, this time in the British Commonwealth, holding the newly created position of principal nursing officer of Jamaica. Nowhere else in the Commonwealth had there been such an office. Here was a Barbadian nurse in the top nursing position, principal nursing officer, in the largest island of the English-speaking Caribbean, Jamaica. It bears repeating that this was no small feat, considering the insularity of the islands. More importantly, it attested to the character of this woman: Nita's lack of pretentiousness and simplicity of demeanour combined with her high principles and standards made her a perfect candidate for that position, apart from the fact that she was a most able public health nurse, nursing tutor and nursing administrator – the three major areas of nursing were already her forte.

During her tenure as principal nursing officer, Nita, forever a mentor and with great foresight, was instrumental in sending five senior nurses to the United States, despite their resistance, to obtain their degree in nursing (even though she herself did not yet have a degree), as she saw them as future leaders in nursing. She gave as her reason the fact that "we in the area, as you know, are not appreciative of degrees as far as nurses' training. And to get them out for the future, you had to start then . . ." This action exemplified Nita's vision and approach. She saw the need to develop future nursing leaders for the West Indies, and the essential value of such education for these younger women in order to assume leadership roles for their people in the many islands.

Nita spoke highly of an American nurse, Janet Thompson, the first nursing advisor with Pan-American Health Organization (PAHO) of the World Health Organization (WHO) for the Caribbean region. They collaborated on the issue of reciprocity of nursing education in the region, where nurses would be able to move freely from one island to another to work, depending on the need. Nita commented: "You were preparing medical students who went to work throughout the area, but nursing was still compartmentalized. The problems of agreeing to that then, as it stood, were obvious because there was no rationalization of training, there was no common basis . . . and Janet was a very wise person. She moved from island to island. She'd always come back and talk about the things we had discussed." Nita acknowledged that she was fortunate and attributed this to two factors. First, although born in Barbados, she had lived in several islands and, with some of her immediate family born in different islands, they were never strictly a one-island family. Second, her experience of being in charge of the School of Public Health made her more aware of the individual islands, their problems and their health needs. Moreover, on the family's return to Barbados from St Croix where they had lived for seven years, they travelled by one of the famous Canadian 'Lady' boats which meant that they stopped at every island. It gave her a clear perception of the islands. She saw this as an asset because travelling of that nature was a rarity for most Caribbean people at that time. And indeed it was. It was only with the growth of UWI and the School of Public Health and Social Welfare preparation that the mixing of the people of the Caribbean islands began.

Nita remained in the position of principal nursing officer longer than any she had previously held – six years. Helen McLean, a teacher of English literature and language, now living in St Kitts, recalled how she first met Nita. She went to study for a year as a mature student at the UCWI in 1958/59, but she did not enjoy living on campus with seventeen- and eighteen-year olds. By pure chance, a friend told her about Nita who lived alone and had a spare bedroom. Nita was most accommodating and welcomed Helen to share her home. They became roommates and found that they had much in common. They liked and laughed at the same things, read the same books, tried out the same recipes and developed a long-lasting friendship. The two shared a bond in cooking and cake decorating and spent many happy hours icing cakes while they lived together. Almost four decades later, Nita, now Dame Nita and governor general of Barbados, had an aide-du-camp who was getting married. Dame Nita made and iced the cake and telephoned Helen in St Kitts to ask her to make the roses to decorate it. Helen made the roses, put them in a box and made her nephew himself carry them (with a multitude of instructions as they were very fragile) from St Kitts to Barbados! Helen recalled that on many occasions Dame Nita would ring her, saying, "I am ringing my consultant, to ask how much colour . . . Is it this much flour? . . . A little softer, I would like it . . ."

Helen quoted Rudyard Kipling's "If" to describe Nita. She continued, "She could associate with the great people of the world and she did, and yet she could talk with the cook or the maid in the hospital and be quite at home with them. To me that was her greatest asset." Helen remembered that after not seeing Nita for fifteen or sixteen years, she had to go to Barbados for knee surgery when her friend was now Dame Nita and governor general. Dame Nita visited her at the hospital and insisted that Helen stay with her at Government House. Helen said to one of the nurses, "Isn't it wonderful how she treats me? She's come here to look for me and to see what I want." The nurse promptly replied, "That is how she treats everybody. Every nurse who ever worked with her, she treats like that."

Nita had the capacity to treat everyone she met as a special and unique human being with dignity, warmth, respect and caring. She had a phenomenal memory for details. When Helen visited Government House and was asked by the butler what she would like to drink, she replied, "Sherry." And before the butler left, Dame Nita said, "Dennis, a sweet sherry. Mrs McLean does not like a dry sherry." Helen was impressed that Dame Nita, after so many years, could remember what she liked and disliked.

Mavis Harney from St Kitts, currently residing in Barbados, met Nita when Mavis and a small group were setting up the Caribbean Nursing Organization (CNO). Mavis is credited as being the brain behind the development of this organization which meets biennially to this day. She also spoke about this endearing feature of Nita – her caring and thoughtfulness. Despite a busy schedule, Nita never forgot people that she met: "One thing about her is that she really was

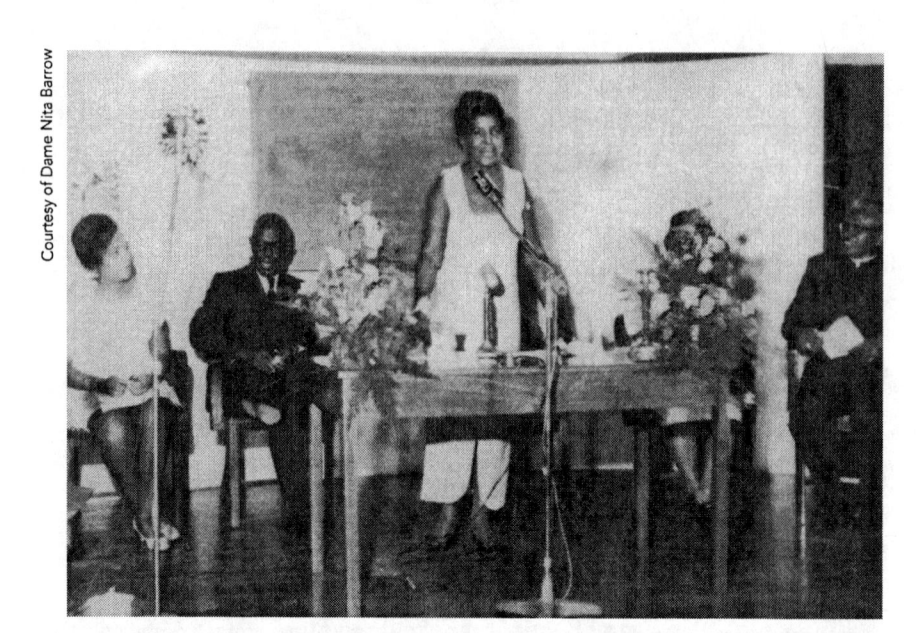

Caribbean Nurses' Organization Meeting, 1968. From left to right, Nita Barrow, Sir Clifford Campbell (governor general of Jamaica), Edna Tulloch (chairman of the Planning Committee), Archbishop Carter, 1968

proud of being a nurse, and always said that once you're a nurse you are always a nurse. And I think this is what made Nita in so many ways stand out . . . We could talk about anything and she really was a very approachable person . . . She always seemed free, so that people could feel free that they could approach her and talk to her . . . I remember the last time was when she had a regional group of nurses who met here in Barbados and she had a reception for them and she included me . . . to see one or two of those people from these islands whom I haven't seen for a long time, because I haven't really been in touch with CNO for a long time."[2]

Practising What She Preached

By 1963 Nita had left for Columbia University, New York, to pursue a bachelor's degree in nursing education, one which she had encouraged so many before her to pursue. She recalled her chief advisor, Miss Eleanor Lambertson saying to her that she "should not have gone in at the bachelor's level. I should have taken the three years [spent] at the University of Toronto and Edinburgh. Just collected the credits and go straight on [to a master's]. I wasn't really interested then. Because it was not the degree you were going after, it was what you knew." They suggested that Nita should stay on for six more months after completing the bachelor's degree, as Nita had taken some master's subjects in addition to her required courses during the two years there. With that additional time, she would be able to get a master's degree. Nita, however, was not interested in doing that because she had taken all the nursing courses, which were her main thrust. Her love of knowledge, her drive to expand her horizons, to broaden her mind, to enrich and share her experiences, these were the pursuits that informed her daily practice and indeed her daily life. These pursuits were of more interest to Nita than obtaining a degree. Her words reflect this desire: "I like to enjoy my experience. I was not working for a degree. I was working for knowledge, so I had the best time in New York than any student."

A change in metropolitan aid to the Caribbean was the major reason for Nita's choice of location of her studies. By the end of the 1960s, the Caribbean had traded its old colonial dependence on Europe for a new dependence on the United States. The decades of the 1950s and 1960s saw a radical transformation of Caribbean economies as North American firms moved into the region on a large scale.[3] The involvement of PAHO in health matters in the Caribbean was therefore inevitable. They took over where Britain left off. The PAHO regional nursing consultant, Janet Thompson, whom Nita knew in her role as principal nurshing officer was instrumental in facilitating Nita's attendance at Columbia University.

Charting a New Course

During the years prior to and during Nita's sojourn in New York, there had been discussion of the need for a survey of all the West Indian schools of nursing. A recurring concern of Nita and others was the inadequate basic preparation of nurses who were taking the public health programme. Future plans for the university post-basic programme and the need for more advanced training for local nurses highlighted how urgent it was to identify deficiencies in the basic training. It was indeed fortunate for Caribbean nursing that in 1963 Nita chose to pursue her studies at Columbia University, at that time universally regarded as *the* university of choice for nursing education. There Nita would meet Helen Mussallem of Canada who was completing her doctorate that year in nursing education. Nita described their encounter: she was having coffee with Dr Eleanor Lambertson and Miss Danson, key nursing educators, and Helen was passing by, having just completed her doctoral defence. Nita said, "I always remember Cathy saying, 'There goes the newest recruit to the noble alley of martyrs' . . . and I rushed up to her [Helen] and said 'Oh! We will need you in the Caribbean. We want to do a study like Canada's. Would you come and join us?'"[4] Needless to say, Helen was most surprised, uttering, "I am sorry, you will have to wait as I have just finished defending my dissertation and we are having coffee." Helen wanted to celebrate, not talk to a stranger. Nita, never one to be deterred, waited for more than an hour until the celebrations were over. Helen approached her and enquired where Nita was from. Helen suggested that Nita herself would be the best person to do such a study because she was a nurse from the Caribbean and pointed out that the Canadian project was so successful because it was done by a Canadian nurse who was familiar with the educational system in Canada. In any event, at that time, Helen was working with the Canadian Nurses' Association as executive director.

Shortly after Nita's return to Jamaica, Janet Thompson approached her on behalf of PAHO to take charge of the project, which was a survey of schools of nursing in the Caribbean. This appointment created history. Helen Mussallem recalled, "It is hard to believe . . . but up to that time WHO had not appointed a national to head a project in his or her own country. In Denmark, you couldn't be a Danish project director; if you were Indian you couldn't head a project in India and likewise in the United States. They said it was not the policy, but we persisted. Janet Thompson, of course, picked it up. She was a wonderful person. I believe, though I can't document this and speak for PAHO, but I think that she [Nita] must have been one of the first nationals to head up any of the PAHO projects in her own country, that was 1962. We are going back a long time . . . Finally, Janet was able to have Nita appointed as the project director with the understanding that I would be a consultant. That was the beginning of our relationship."[5]

This was a relationship that lasted until Dame Nita's death in 1995. The nature and extent of the project, under Nita's leadership, warrants elaboration, as it had far-reaching consequences for the future of nursing education and nursing leadership to the current time.

Setting the Stage for Change

The newly formed Federation of the West Indies in the period between 1958 and 1961 greatly facilitated regional cooperation of both a governmental and nongovernmental nature in nursing. Despite the dissolution of the Federation, the framework was laid for collaborative efforts which have continued to the present time.

On 31 August 1959, a group of senior nursing personnel from the Commonwealth Caribbean met in Barbados to discuss the problems confronting them. This was the first time nursing administrators, nursing educators, and representatives of general nursing councils and nursing associations had ever assembled together. They represented the ten then British territories of Antigua, Barbados, Grenada, Jamaica, Montserrat, St Kitts–Nevis–Anguilla, St Lucia, St Vincent, and Trinidad and Tobago. Although British Guiana, British Honduras and the Bahamas were not a part of the Federation, they were invited to send representatives to the meeting since their nursing education programmes also followed the British pattern.

They met at a time marked by rapid political, educational and socioeconomic change in which much closer relationships were developing among West Indian territories. Under the auspices of the Federal Government of the West Indies, Dr Horace Gillette, federal medical advisor, chaired that historic Conference of Caribbean Nursing Administrators in Barbados. Its terms of reference were to study, compare, and evaluate the nursing needs of the unit territories of the Federation, British Guiana and British Honduras; to discuss the educational requirements and training of nurses; and to discuss the possibility of the establishment of a federal nursing register with reciprocity within the Federation and other countries overseas. Hopes were held high by all, medical as well as nursing personnel, for finding solutions to the many problems facing nursing in the territories. In her speech at the opening ceremonies, Nita, then principal nursing officer for Jamaica, expressed such sentiments eloquently:

We are therefore grateful for this Conference and welcome it as an opportunity to look at our needs realistically and we hope in a fashion which leaves us unafraid. We have to consider the light of modern trends because changes which are taking place in our own profession like that of many others cannot be kept back any more than the tides of the sea . . . We hope at the end of this period which we share we shall have a much clearer vision not of the problems, because they bow us down, but of some of the solutions towards which we can work and go forward in that spirit into what appears to be a challenging and exciting future . . .[6]

It was in such a mood of enthusiasm that the whole spectrum of issues confronting nurses in the region was explored through subcommittees, with subsequent recommendations. Manpower needs, socioeconomic matters, postgraduate training, the establishment of professional organizations, reciprocity of registration, and the training of student nurses were only a few of the topics discussed. It cannot be sufficiently emphasized that only training recognized by a body external to the region, namely the General Nursing Council for England and Wales, was accepted by all the islands' authorities as equipping a nurse to practise her profession outside her home territory. Graduates of schools that had not obtained such recognition were normally required to undergo additional preparation in order to validate their certificates. Since there was no regulatory body in the region responsible for interisland standards, improvements in nursing programmes had to be made in order to secure their complete or partial recognition by the General Nursing Council for England and Wales, regardless of whether or not they were called for by the needs of the territories themselves.

The subcommittee that addressed the education of student nurses was in agreement that it was desirable to have a minimum educational standard for all territories, and suggested the designing of an educational test that would accommodate varying standards. It advocated encouraging prospective candidates to continue beyond the school leaving certificate by the provision of courses in English, arithmetic and the health sciences at a more advanced level in order to better prepare them for further training.[7]

Evolving from this conference was a steering committee of eight members, who were as representative as possible of the area as a whole. Its task was to carry out a searching review of the recommendations of the conference and, later, to function in the role of an advisory committee to a proposed federal nursing officer.

The steering committee met in Trinidad in 1961 to carry out its task as envisioned by the conference group. It recommended a survey of schools of nursing in the territories in order to ascertain the educational standards and needs of the area. Despite the demise of the political federation in 1962, the PAHO/WHO nursing consultants, Janet Thompson and Verna Huffman (now Huffman Splane), who was the PAHO/WHO nursing consultant to the federal government and stationed in Trinidad at that time, gave much assistance to the group in their quest for international aid for the evaluation of the educational programmes in the area and kept the spark alive. The dissolution of Federation brought many changes: two of the islands became independent states; some achieved full or partial self-government; and others were moving towards independence. Consequently, the consent, help and cooperation of each of the thirteen governments had to be sought separately. In 1963 the plan that had been formulated by the steering committee was submitted to PAHO/WHO. This led to the development of a project addressing nursing education, beginning with a survey of the twenty-three schools of nursing, including British Guiana, British Honduras and the Bahamas.

REGIONAL LEADERSHIP

By 1964 it was inevitable that Nita would be seconded from her position as principal nursing officer in Jamaica to WHO for three years to head that major project. This was another first – Nita was the first PAHO/WHO nurse from the Caribbean. Dr Helen Mussallem, executive director of the Canadian Nurses' Association, was also seconded as a short-term consultant to the project in 1965. With her considerable experience and expertise, she rendered extremely valuable assistance to the project throughout the stages of development and execution. Helen came to the Caribbean for about six weeks each year for the first two years of the project. Nita also brought with her a thorough knowledge of the problems as well as a rich background and education. Nita and Janet Thompson, on whom Nita lavished praise for her sensitivity and understanding, spent the first few months in defining how they would carry out this project. They based their approach on the Canadian survey *Spotlight on Nursing Education* which Nita found most interesting. The real challenge was to use nurses from the countries involved to make up teams. The Board of Review was the first to be set up with senior nurses from the islands, then that board assisted in determining the number of 'visitors' required to go with Nita, as project officer, into each territory. These were the survey teams which consisted of Nita and one regional visitor. Four phases of the project were envisioned:

1. Collecting of factual information by the survey teams;
2. Evaluating this information for the purpose of future planning by the Board of Review;
3. Formulating plans for the improvement of nursing education at a nursing education seminar to be held after completion of the survey and the evaluation;
4. Implementing the plans, which would be dependent on the interest of the individual governments.

The eight members of the steering committee which had recommended the survey served on the advisory committee to the project. They formed a board of review for the evaluation of the schools of nursing in the thirteen territories.[8]

As head of the project, Nita had to visit each territory to convince the various governments that such a project was necessary and to get their cooperation and their commitment to a certain part of the funding. They were asked to release one of their senior nurses to travel to a neighbouring territory as a member of the survey team; provide accommodation for the visiting regional visitor, and internal transportation at the time of the survey visit to their territory; and, on request, give permission for senior nursing personnel and others to attend the meetings of the Board of Review and nursing education seminars. For the three years that Nita was based in Antigua, the government provided the project with an office and a secretary, some supplies, free postage and also internal transportation. Antigua had been selected as the base because it was in the middle of the chain and central to all the islands. Nita could not be assigned to Barbados, as it was her country of origin, nor to Jamaica, as she had been recruited from her position there. This position of project director would refine Nita's political and negotiating skills, if they ever needed refining. As she observed, "The minister of health, you started with him. Because you had to be political really first and we often met with the chief minister or the prime minister." These encounters enhanced her profile throughout the Caribbean and internationally.

While the survey was being conducted in a territory, seven hours of meetings were allotted for senior nurses and senior government officials, such as medical officers of health. The survey was presented to them and they were able to discuss the administration and evaluation of the exercise. Nita's role and responsibilities were vast. Strong organizational abilities were required as well as excellent interpersonal and political skills in dealing with government ministers, matrons, members of boards of institutions controlling schools of nursing, teaching staff, nurses and medical associations, general nursing councils, and other nursing personnel. Briefing through correspondence, writing the many reports connected with the project as well as establishing and maintaining procedures and records were but a few of the manifold responsibilities that Nita carried out with aplomb, diplomacy and tact.

The criteria used in evaluating the schools were those utilized by Mussallem in the Canadian survey of nursing education programmes, but adapted and modified for use in the English-speaking Caribbean. After a careful study of each of the twenty-three programmes, the Board of Review reached the conclusion that only one school met the agreed criteria. Each school was presented with a document indicating both its strengths and the areas that needed improvement. Because only Nita, one regional visitor and Helen conducted all twenty-three surveys in the thirteen islands, Helen laid down a few very strict rules, explaining, "I knew that it was my responsibility to indoctrinate them." Helen had many anecdotes about their experiences during the survey. She recalled that "Rule number one was that absolutely no evenings were to be spent in any activity other than writing the report, discussions etcetera, relative to the relevant survey. Because if you surveyed all day, you had to write at night in order to get all done in one week. One week, we were in Antigua where Nita was headquartered. I noticed some unusual activities, maids and porters were busy delivering small and large packages which Nita put on top of the fridge. By Thursday, I was becoming really suspicious and said to Nita, 'I hope that you are not having guests before we finish on Saturday.' No reply. You didn't push Nita, no matter what your authority. While we were writing the report at Nita's place in the Sugar Mills Flats in Antigua, activity increased as Nita divided her time between receiving parcels and writing her share of the report. At 7 p.m. I was still busy writing when guests arrived. Nita had recruited the assistance of maids, waiters and friends and together they put on the best party with about sixty people – the governor of the island, the medical officers and their wives, and nurses. She had them do this very subtly and I was furious and I said, 'Nita, I said no parties we have got to write this report.' Nita replied, 'I've written my part of the report and you've done yours.' She couldn't see why we had to be serious the night before we had to present the report. Then we put the report together and took it over to my flat and I joined in the fun because I thought, 'That is enough of that!' "

The nurses who came as members of the Board of Review met in the garage of the hotel in Antigua. While the accommodation was not satisfactory, it was the only place available for meeting. When there was a tropical downpour the meeting had to be rescheduled as they could not hear each other because of the sound of the rain. Helen observed that it was "quite a contrast thirteen years later when the regional body was set up and we met at the Holiday Inn. In Canada, we had a suite at the Château Laurier and in Antigua we met in an open garage – quite a contrast."[9] Despite this, Helen also observed that "the quality of both groups involved was, in my opinion, equal. They were just as good as the Canadian people."

In association with this project, four seminars were held in various territories. The first two were directly concerned with the execution of the survey, review of the survey findings, final assessment of the schools, and planning for the future. Participants were primarily senior administrative nursing personnel. One of the recommendations of the second seminar held in Antigua in 1965 advised members of the teaching staff of the nursing schools to hold a seminar "to work out a curriculum suitable for the preparation of nurses of all categories". Consequently, the third seminar on nursing education in January 1966 brought together those responsible for nursing education programmes in the area, and guidelines were developed for planning basic nursing programmes appropriate to the Caribbean. The fourth seminar was held in Guyana in 1968, to evaluate the progress in improvement of nursing education in the countries involved and to assist the teaching staff in curriculum development. PAHO/WHO advisors provided assistance throughout these seminars, in addition to Dr Helen Mussallem. A number of workshops and seminars were held for nursing staff during the survey. Marie Matthews, a PAHO/WHO consultant based in Barbados, conducted ongoing ward administration courses for ward sisters from all the islands. The Queen Elizabeth Hospital had recently opened and had very good facilities, so ongoing ward administration courses were provided under the PAHO team.

The third phase of the project – the formulation of future plans – was entrusted to a nursing education seminar, to be held after completion of the survey and the final evaluation. This took place after the last meeting of the Board of Review in Antigua in August 1965. The participants included members of the Board of Review and seven senior nursing officers from territories not represented on the board; government officials representing finance, planning, public health administration and hospital administration; members of the faculty of UWI, including a member of the staff of the Institute of Education, of the Department of Government, and of the Faculty of Medicine; and PAHO/WHO staff, including advisors in planning and in public health administration and four nursing advisors.

The seminar was to study the results of the evaluation of the schools of nursing presented by the Board of Review with a view to improving nursing services by raising the standard of nursing education, and to planning for the future development of nursing. Four major recommendations resulted from the seminar. The first called for two categories of nurses to meet the needs of nursing services; the second addressed the need to improve the basic nursing education programmes as recommended by the Board of Review and to develop a suitable curriculum. The third recommendation advised that steps be taken to set up a regional nursing body with a specified mandate and specific representation. The final recommendation concerned the Advanced Nursing Education Programme. The UWI representatives from the Institute of Education and the government outlined plans for the development of such a programme to prepare nurse tutors and administrators.[10]

Nursing Advisor

The seminal Conference of Caribbean Nursing Administrators in 1959 had written a charter for the future direction of nursing and nursing education in the Commonwealth Caribbean. It laid the foundation for the establishment of a regional nursing body as recommended. The regional nursing body was envisioned as being responsible for accreditation of schools, offering advice and assistance in improving standards of nursing education, and conducting periodic evaluation of programmes. The recommendation was endorsed at the nursing education seminars held in Jamaica in 1966 and Guyana in 1968, and further discussed in Dominica at a seminar organized by PAHO/WHO in 1969. In that year, at the first conference of Caribbean health ministers, a resolution was passed endorsing the establishment of such a regional nursing body.

As a result of this continuing interest, a meeting was sponsored by the Commonwealth Foundation which convened in Barbados in April 1970, under the chairmanship of Ena Walters, matron of the Queen Elizabeth Hospital. Ena also created nursing history as she was the first local nurse to be appointed matron in Barbados. The Commonwealth Foundation gave a grant of money to facilitate bringing together a group of twelve senior nurses from the Commonwealth Caribbean with two Canadian and two British nurses as consultants and two resource persons from the Caribbean. One of these resource persons was Nita Barrow who, on completion of the survey, continued to work with PAHO/WHO in the Caribbean as a nursing advisor. Others were Janet Thompson and Marie Matthews, PAHO/WHO nursing advisors; Dr Helen Mussallem, executive director of the Canadian Nurses Association; and Verna Huffman, principal nursing officer, Canada. The group appointed a steering committee of six members, with four alternates, to continue working on the development of the Regional Nursing Body. The group also requested that a resurvey of schools of nursing be conducted in order to provide the regional body with up-to-date information on nursing education in the region. They decided to request the governments to approve such a resurvey and recommended that PAHO/WHO be asked to conduct the resurvey. Resolutions to that effect were incorporated in the final report which was submitted to the second conference of health ministers of the Commonwealth Caribbean in April 1970. The conference of ministers agreed in principle with both the establishment of a regional nursing body and the request for a resurvey of nursing schools. The resurvey was started in 1970 and completed in 1971.[11] Nita was again entrusted with that task, and it was deemed simple by Nita, "because you just checked up on things that had been done and emphasized, and then the final report".

Although Nita had garnered vast knowledge and experience in nursing education, nursing service and public health through her varied roles in the Caribbean, she was not content to focus only on nursing. Her interests always encompassed the broader realm of human concerns. She had long worked with the YWCA and also with the World Council of Churches (WCC). She had been appointed associate director of the Christian Medical Commission (CMC) in 1970 while still on contract at PAHO. However, when she was offered that position, she continued to supervise the Caribbean project to its completion in 1971. In 1976, a notable year for her, she became director of the CMC and president of the World YWCA. Two major achievements – the first black president of the worldwide YWCA, and the first woman, and a black, to head the CMC. How did Nita achieve this?

President of the World YWCA

The World YWCA unites twenty-five million women working in ninety-two countries to achieve common social justice for women by increasing their participation in social, economic and political activities at all levels of society. The YWCA works to achieve its mission through programmes that focus on improving the health and safety of women and girls; recognizing and valuing diversity; and improving women's economic and political power. Nita's own goals and activities were so consistent with the ideals of the YWCA that it seemed inevitable that she would be increasingly involved with and committed to that organization. From as far back as the mid-forties when Nita was in Trinidad en route to Canada to study public health nursing at the University of Toronto, she had become a member of the newly formed YWCA through the secretary of the YWCA, Phyllis Haslam. In Toronto, she became an associate member of that YWCA and used the facilities there from time to time. When she came to Jamaica to do her fieldwork in public health, she lived in the YWCA hostel. It was at one of the YWCA Monday afternoon lectures that she and Carmen Lusan of Jamaica were to meet and a long-lasting friendship ensued. Nita was soon a member of the board of the Kingston YWCA. Carmen eventually became the first Caribbean woman to be general secretary of the YWCA of Jamaica. At the time, she was already in a secure job in the civil service and was reluctant to apply for the post but, as she said, "Eventually I decided to do it with [Nita's] encouragement. That is the kind of person that she is. To make one feel with more confidence than one has and so I began to get ready for that. In 1947 I took the first course in England as I was not trained as a social worker."[12] Carmen stayed in that position for nine years, living in residence at the YWCA. This afforded her more opportunities to see Nita who lived there for a while. They eventually bought and shared a house when Nita was matron of UCHWI and this further cemented the friendship.

Nita sat on many YWCA committees and eventually on the Island Council, the policy-making body. It was a fortunate coincidence for Nita that when she went to do the sister tutor course in England in 1950, the World YWCA Council was holding its quadrennial meeting in Lebanon. The YWCA in Jamaica could not afford to send a delegate and since Nita was on the council, it was suggested that, if she could take time off from her studies, she would be an appropriate person to go to Lebanon as a representative of the Jamaica YWCA. It was Nita's first venture into an international YWCA meeting and she made a most favourable impression on all who met her. This eventually led to her becoming the first woman from the English-speaking Caribbean to be elected to the executive committee of the World Council. The worldwide YWCA had a nominating committee which was briefed to recruit members from all the geographical regions of the world. Up to 1950 the YWCA was largely comprised of European and North American members. The leadership had become anxious that the council should include representatives from all over the world. As a member of the executive committee, Nita had to travel to Geneva for World Council meetings and every four years to whichever country was to be the host of the quadrennial meeting. For part of that time, Nita was also chairman of the Caribbean Area Committee with primary responsibility for the YWCA in the region. After World War II had ended, many of the associations were floundering because they had been started by expatriates who were then returning to their own countries. The Caribbean Area Committee of the YWCA was formed in 1957. Carmen Lusan was later appointed area secretary. Nita was the first chairperson to ensure that representatives from many of the islands would be members of the committee. She was suitably qualified to hold that chair as she was not only a council member of the

World YWCA, which meant that she travelled extensively, but also her then role as project director with PAHO/WHO required her to travel throughout the Caribbean.

In 1975 Nita was elected president at the World Council meeting in Vancouver, making her the first black woman to be elected to that post. She would be elected again in Athens in 1979, thus serving two terms. One of Nita's many gifts was the ability to forge a unity between her salaried work and her voluntary role. She was particularly adept at combining work and volunteer activities, for whenever she was travelling in her official role as PAHO/WHO advisor in the region she would seize the opportunity to visit the YWCA in the various islands. The same held true for her commitments worldwide. Wherever she attended a meeting, she would also find time to visit the YWCA in that city or country. Her thrust was always for social justice and she saw that by empowering women in many areas of all societies this could be achieved. It was only fitting that in 1976 the first university to confer on her a degree of Doctor of Laws was UWI.

DIRECTOR OF THE CHRISTIAN MEDICAL COMMISSION

The YWCA was not Nita's only volunteer activity. Her interest in the broader realm of health care and her Christian beliefs led her to become involved with the WCC. This worldwide organization seeks to promote the unity of the Church and humankind. The WCC is a fellowship of Anglican, Protestant, Orthodox and other non-Roman Catholic Christians in over one hundred countries and with over four hundred million members. It stands for ecumenism and the strengthening of ties in the whole Christian Church community. It is active in international affairs, provides help to developing countries, joins in international efforts to relieve suffering caused by wars and natural disasters and assists in the resettlement of refugees. Through its Commission of the Churches on International Affairs, WCC is accredited to the United Nations (UN) Economic and Social Council as a nongovernmental organization. Its headquarters are at the Ecumenical Centre in Geneva.[13]

In 1968 Nita was invited by the WCC to attend a conference in Tübingen, Germany, at which the role of the Christian church in health care would be addressed. Two earlier conferences had been held in Tubingen to re-examine the theological basis of the churches' concern for health. The need to make a systematic attempt to understand Christian thinking and action in the churches' healing ministry, within the ecumenical movement, resulted in the formation of a new CMC. The mandate of the commission was to set up and develop means for sustained enquiry, description and reflection concerning connections between health, being human, the community and the Kingdom of God. The CMC was also concerned with the theological and medical aspects of fundamental questions of health and wholeness and the "church's healing ministry".[14]

Nita was invited to become a member of the new commission which would be finalized at this conference. She accepted the invitation and, as a member or a commissioner from its inception, would volunteer her rich experience in nursing education, nursing service and community health garnered through the years in Jamaica and the Caribbean through her involvement with the PAHO/WHO project.

There was a strategy behind Nita's invitation to that conference in Tubingen. She had been invited not only for her advocacy role in the teaching of primary health care and her nursing expertise. The secretary general of the WCC was Dr Philip Potter, a lifelong friend of Nita from the days when she was assistant instructor at the School of Public Health in Jamaica and he was a theological student. He, together with Dr James MacGilvray, the director of the CMC, and others thought that Nita would be a valuable addition to their staff in helping them to implement the new CMC strategies. They wanted the other commissioners of the WCC to have the opportunity to meet Nita and possibly consider her for a position on the commission. Their plan worked. In 1972 Nita was appointed associate director of the WCC's CMC in Geneva,[15] a city she knew well, having visited it every year since 1957 as a member of the executive of the World YWCA.

In June 1976 Nita became a member of the staff of the CMC as the first woman to become director of the commission. She was to serve in that position until 1981. During that period, innovative programmes of health care, now designated "Primary Health Care", were identified and formed part of the worldwide concept enunciated by WHO as "Health for All by the Year 2000". Nita explained that the job of the CMC was to help local people to upgrade their health care by using indigenous remedies and, in many cases, incorporating traditional healers such as witch doctors. In other words, the intent was to introduce the concept of primary health care by taking positive preventive measures in terms of food, water and sanitation before going to the doctor, even if one were available. Nita was always an ardent advocate of participatory community involvement through utilizing the basic knowledge and skills of members of the community. She noted:

We were like brokers looking for worthwhile projects to fund and learning all the while: for instance, that the Inuits of America and the Aborigines of Australia had their own forms of alternative health care and that these could be incorporated into more modern methods . . . Teach them the basic skills of health care and only the very ill will need to go to hospitals and thus the cost to the country is decreased . . . In countries with traditional healers we brought them into meetings where their knowledge could be used . . . In Belize and Guyana we trained traditional birth attendants chosen by the community itself. They were therefore known and trusted . . .[16]

Nita's philosophy embraced the twin notions of responsibility and self-reliance for individuals as well as communities. Indeed, her life exemplified both these qualities. Dr Philip Potter observed in 1986 that

Nita has not only excelled professionally in her pioneering work in health service in Jamaica, in the Caribbean through WHO, and in the world as Director of the Christian Medical Commission of the World Council of Churches, but she has also taught us all through her example to care for the whole person and for all the people . . . Nita is here and everywhere, sharing her wit and wisdom, her beautiful spirit and her bountiful knowledge, and her embodiment of health, healing, and wholeness. Nita is indeed the dame woman in her all-embracing love, bearing and affirming our humanity in all its fullness.[17]

Long before primary health care became a catch phrase, Nita, as director of the CMC, ensured that it was truly practised. Her role as director made it possible for her to travel to all parts of the world and, in particular, the developing countries. Moreover, since the work of the CMC and WHO was complementary in terms of the promotion of basic health services, her travels facilitated greater liaison between the two organizations. The director of WHO, with a staff of twelve hundred, approached Nita with a proposal to form an official joint standing committee comprised of members of the small staff of the CMC and staff members of WHO. Nita is said to have remarked immediately, "I feel like David confronted by Goliath." And the director's response was, "Nita, you forget that I am a Lutheran minister's son and I early learned what happened to Goliath!" That partnership led to the WHO international conference on primary health care at Alma Ata, Russia, in September 1978. The historic statement on "Health for All by the Year 2000" resulted from that conference.[18]

The annual meeting of the CMC in 1977 was held at the Royal Holloway College, Egham, just outside London, and it was a highly unusual one in the history of the CMC. The term of the original commission had expired at the same time as the fifth assembly of the WCC, held in Nairobi at the close of 1975. A new commission had been appointed in the interim, and consequently, for many members of the newly constituted commission, it was their first opportunity to share directly in the work of the CMC. Most importantly, Nita had been appointed director of the commission ten months earlier and it was the first annual meeting she would attend in her new capacity. However, the most unusual aspect of the gathering was the presence of the other four WCC commissions of the Programme Unit on Justice and Service, also meeting at the same site. They were the Commission of Inter-Church Aid, Refugee and World Service; the Commission of the Churches' Participation in Development; the Commission of the Churches on International Affairs; and the Programme to Combat Racism. In order to promote greater coordination among themselves and their activities, the five subunits had planned to hold their meetings concurrently that year. Their common theme was for a just, participatory and sustainable society. Central to all these units and their programmes was the struggle for human dignity and social justice. The world at that time was shaken by a number of global crises: a major food crisis, a monetary system in disarray, economic systems and theories under challenge, systematic injustice, scarcity of resources, environmental deterioration, and increasing malnutrition were threatening the survival of mankind. Nita's sensitivity to these concerns were noted in her first director's report:

From its very beginning, the CMC has been concerned with the question of health care and social justice – the most comprehensive ethical issue in health care for the churches. In the search for a new social order, and as the church tries to find its role in this search, the questions of health and health care provision come back again and again to the interrelated dynamics of justice, participation and sustainability. In many parts of the world, land tenure, employment opportunities, the basic conveniences of water and sanitation, the capacity of the rural sector to feed itself and other pressures of social injustice constitute the gravest public health problems. This looms even larger than the well known distributive injustice in the health care services. Many are still deprived of a reasonable chance to have a healthy life by the decision-makers. Furthermore, present patterns exclude the vast majority of people from participating in any way in their concern for health. They do not have an opportunity to identify their needs, to express them or to establish the priorities. They have no share in the process of planning to meet those needs, and they are given no say or responsibility in the administration and control of the health care system. The whole dimension of people's participation is so crucial to the justice and sustainability of the social system as it relates to health. A healthy society cannot be sustained unless everyone is involved and responsible. Sustainability is also closely tied to the matter of technology for healthy living. It is essential that a people of a given place be able to master and sustain the technology utilized in health care, in agriculture and nutrition, in the development of water supplies, energy and sanitation, and in the training and administration of those who work in the sphere of health, agriculture, and community development.[19]

In August 1980 Nita decided to take her 'retirement' to return to Barbados, and submitted her resignation as director of CMC. This came as a shock to many who had been hoping that her occasional hints about "going while still appreciated" and "time to move on" were simply her brand of dry humour. However, consistent with her belief in the need for change and renewal – which allowed many different institutions, organizations and groups to benefit from her unique talents and qualities over the years – Nita resolved to leave CMC and Geneva before the end of the term of the current commission. Her resignation was accepted with a feeling of desolation among staff and commissioners. In its tribute to her, the *CMC News* expressed deep gratitude to her for her inspiration and guidance, for her vision of the commission's role, for her unique way of relating to and with people, and for her unwavering devotion to health and human development. The *News* aptly observed that even her decision to leave reflected those qualities. As a parting gift on the eve of her departure as director of the CMC, Nita contributed some of her thoughts on nursing to *Contact*, the organization's monthly publication. A woman clearly ahead of her time, all that she had to say almost two decades ago still resonates with truth today. Her major thrust, as always, was to advocate again for the provision of basic health care for all rather than quality care only for the few and flexibility in the role of the nurse in primary health care. She expounded:

Part of the nurse's role in PHC [primary health care] may also be to re-examine people's health needs as well as the causes of ill health. In this, nurses will need to be prepared to be the learners from teachers less skilled and sophisticated than themselves. They will need to admit that the cures of ill health go beyond the bacteria they see under their microscopes and that the majority of them have their origins in such factors as poor housing, and sanitation, lack of potable water, unemployment and lack of adequate food, among others... What nurses must accept, therefore, is a role which can vary according to the needs of the situation. *The nurse must be willing to learn what is really needed and then to share that knowledge appropriate to the time and place with others, thus enabling them to safely carry out caring and curing tasks and functions, and enhancing their role within, and in the eyes of the community.*[20]

Nita argued for the value and centrality of positive attitudes and interpersonal relationships of the nurse – both of which she exemplified. She observed that all actions would have little or no effect if the teacher were not accepted and trusted by the community as someone who cared and who understood them and their needs. Unless people felt that the nurse or caring person was prepared to discuss their own perceptions of their needs and, through dialogue, arrive at a mutually acceptable solution, treatment, advice and teaching would have very little long-term effect. Her love of nursing was evident as she implored the profession to examine itself. Primary health care was posed as the means through which the caring aspect could be restored to nursing. She challenged nursing to consider how it could best continue to grow as a caring, sharing profession, be concerned with people and their needs, and at the same time promote this growth by giving some of the knowledge, skills and prerogatives of the profession to colleagues with less training and to the wider community.[21] Those challenges still face nursing today.

ADULT EDUCATION FOR WOMEN

Yet another of Nita's activities was her involvement in adult education. This interest starts with Roby Kidd, a well-respected and greatly admired Canadian, and an acknowledged guru of adult education, who was chairman of the Department of Adult Education, Ontario Institute for Studies in Education, Toronto, from 1966 until his death in 1982. His eminence in the field nationally and internationally through his involvement with a myriad of organizations dedicated to adult education for the underprivileged is renowned. He was the founder of the International Council of Adult Education (ICAE) in 1973 and served as its first secretary general. Roby's passion was exploring ways to educate adults and to provide access to learning opportunities which could emancipate women and men in all parts of the world. The notion of education as a component of development had, for the past two decades, been the goals of international development of organizations such as the United Nations Educational, Scientific and Cultural Organization (UNESCO) and the World Bank. A measure of the man was that as early as 1972, he was commissioned by the International Development Research Centre, Ottawa, to conduct an international enquiry singlehandedly on Education for Development.[22]

At the seventh annual meeting of the ICAE in Finland in 1979, it was agreed that the priorities of adult education would be on activities that promote economic and social justice and world peace. Astute as he was, Roby recognized that the ICAE priorities dovetailed with the concept of primary health care. His travels throughout the world, and in the developing countries in particular, provided him with great insight into the cultures and lives of the less privileged peoples of the world. It comes as no surprise to learn that, on a subsequent visit to Geneva, Roby encouraged Nita to become involved with the work of ICAE, now that they were moving into countries such as China and Vietnam. He was aware of Nita's strong international advocacy role of primary health care and that she would be supportive of ICAE's involvement in those less developed countries. Initially hesitant to become involved, claiming her lack of knowledge and experience in this field, Nita told how Roby Kidd had persuaded her: "He said, 'You have been teaching nursing for fifteen years, you are an adult educator . . . Don't tell me that you're not doing adult education: you have been doing it most of your professional life.' . . . When I got into it I found that what we're talking about is the whole role of educating people for life and for living, but literacy comes first."

The activities of the two organizations were a logical blend. Indeed, Nita's and Roby's personalities as well as their philosophical beliefs and approaches to people shared common strands. Roby gave his life in the service of relating continuous education of adults to the world condition. He saw adult education as enhancing the human potential which would lead to justice, better communication between cultures, improved cooperation and, ultimately, towards peace.[23] Nita's beliefs about nursing and primary health care mirrored these principles. She was invited to the next ICAE annual meeting in France in 1982 while still president of the World YWCA. Sadly, Roby died just shortly before that conference.

Women had been doing much of the work of ICAE over the years but none were present at the decision-making level. Nita made it clear that she would be lobbying for a more visible role for them. She had been asked to assist with the women's programme and to address and lead the seminar on the role of women within the context of the theme of the conference, which was "Towards an Authentic Development: The Role of Adult Education". It was to Nita's sheer consternation that she was elected president at that conference. A sole woman once more among twenty-three men. Adamant as she was about changes in the secondary role of women in that organization, one of her objectives during her term of office was to ensure a higher profile for women on the ICAE executive. Two others were to bring women from all parts of the world closer together and to reorganize the management structure of the ICAE so that it could become more decentralized from Toronto, its original home base. To facilitate this, Nita formed an advisory committee with the objective of providing wider participation in the decision-making process. A new managerial structure was created that allowed for six regional associations of ICAE in Africa, the Arab countries, Asia and South Pacific, Latin America, the Caribbean, and Europe. As was usual in most organizations at that time, the power structure of ICAE was male dominated with women, who often felt uninvolved and inadequate, as support staff. Nita was good for the morale of women, especially at council meetings where males were in the majority and tended to dominate the discussion. By the end of Nita's second and final term as president in 1990, there were four women vice presidents in ICAE.[24]

Nita provided strong, firm, democratic and moral leadership. As president, she travelled widely and visited Muslim countries and China, among many others. Her continued interest in equality for women and the principles of primary health care made it possible for her to observe how these were implemented. Nita's style of speaking was lucid and firm, yet gentle and caring. Her nonthreatening manner made her points of view appear reasonable and favourable to all who heard her and she was respected for them. During Nita's stewardship, the ICAE had made a contribution to the worldwide interest in literacy as a means of all people developing a true sense of their self-worth. Nita managed to secure funds to assist representatives to attend conferences, including some of the graduates of ICAE as well as other literacy programmes worldwide. The climax of Nita's association with ICAE was the provision of funds for the Dame Nita Barrow Award, on an annual basis, to recognize and support regional and national adult education organizations that made a significant contribution towards the empowerment of women in the adult education field.

Nita's international stature was growing with these varied high-profile roles and activities – often she was the only woman among men. She had the further distinction in 1985 of being appointed to serve as one of the Commonwealth Group of Eminent Persons to South Africa to broker the transformation there. She was once more the only woman in a seven-member group. She brought special insight in health matters to the high-powered male team who journeyed to South Africa to investigate whether any possibilities existed for negotiation and dialogue between the government and the anti-apartheid groups. The fact-finding mission met over seven months with Nelson Mandela, Oliver Tambo, Alan Boesek, Archbishop Tutu, government officials and local community leaders, all attempting to find a peaceful solution. She was the first foreign visitor allowed to see Nelson Mandela in prison and many credit her compelling personal power with helping to sway South African president F.W. de Klerk to free Mandela. Sir Shridath Ramphal, chancellor of UWI, who was also one of the eminent persons who went to South Africa, recounted that Nita was

always on the side of justice, always on the side of people. For me there is a special bond. Out of the tremendous contributions she made to the freedom in Southern Africa . . . Nita Barrow was one of the first persons from outside South Africa . . . to see Nelson Mandela in Pollsmoor prison. It was a beginning that was to pave the way for freedom and justice and a new beginning for South Africa. That was the dimension of this woman's life and work and reach.[25]

As usual, Nita's life continued at the same hectic pace that would weary others. She seemed to have an extraordinary capacity to embrace a host of activities. In the same year that she went to South Africa, she was invited to convene the nongovernmental organization's conference, Forum '85, UN Decade of Women held in Nairobi, Kenya. Nita was passionate about the advancement of the status of women, Caribbean women in particular, and was able to achieve much for their cause through her warm and unpretentious manner. She observed, in her usual humorous fashion, that when she was asked to head the organizing committee to mark the end of the UN Decade for Women, she agreed, saying, " 'So long as I haven't got to raise funds, so long as I don't have to live in New York, and so long as I don't have any meetings.' How often can you get conned? So you won't have to raise funds, everybody will help. Everybody. Any time you hear that term 'everybody', say no thanks. Everybody becomes nobody when you get there!" Nita had to move to New York for eighteen months, maintaining a full-time office to coordinate the various planning committees located in Nairobi, Geneva, Vienna and New York, organizing fund raising, as well as working closely with the governments involved. Nita, just as she did when at ICAE, used funds raised to help delegates attend the forum. The funds were also used for pre-conference consultations, regional meetings and for questionnaires sent out so that women around the world could indicate what they wanted included in the agenda.

Seventeen thousand five hundred women of every race and creed, urban and rural, rich and poor, young and old, and a few men, attended the conference, with 1,250 workshops held over the ten-day period. It was one of the largest UN gatherings ever, so much so that accommodation was a problem. It was partially solved by the use of university dormitories. It took tremendous political skill, supreme patience and tact and low-keyed but magnetic personal charisma to mediate between a prickly Kenyan government and a volatile gathering of these nongovernmental delegates.

Dame Nita was of the opinion that it was important that the women be able to talk:

We had women of every dissident group you can think of. We had not only the Palestinian women from the camps, we had the Israeli from Israel . . . we had the women from Eritrea and the women from Ethiopia, with Ethiopia saying there is no such country as Eritrea, you can't have Eritrean women, there are none. And we'd go through every country, any country that had two sets of governments and many forms of protest groups. We had them all because we did not register countries, we registered women. We did not register political entities, we registered women. We had three slogans for them. Any time you got into a confrontation, you were to say, how did this affect me as a woman? Second, any time that one person was speaking, you listened so that they would listen to you. And the third was when you listened, you tried to hear.[26]

She was able to coax warring factions of women to meet face to face and talk informally. They were there to share and a Peace Tent was set up where problems could be sorted out, for example, a dispute which inevitably arose between the Israeli and Palestinian delegates. Her sense of humour was evident in crisis situations. "When there weren't enough rooms to hold workshops or meetings, women used the facilities of nature: shady trees and grassy lawns. Even the well-known American feminist Betty Friedan – now far less strident than in her earlier days – was contented to hold her workshops under a tree . . . We said to her before we left New York, 'Well, Betty, you'll have to pick a tree!' In fun! Betty picked a tree and every day at noon she had her seminar under the tree. She rushed in one day to the office where, you know, you had one hundred and one things going on, she said to me, 'Nita someone has gone and taken away my tree.' And I said, 'Where have they taken it?' Honestly, and it is the only thing, somebody says to you they've taken it away, you say, 'But where they've taken it?' 'Oh! No! No!' she said. 'The handicapped are meeting under my tree.' I said, 'Find another.' She said, 'The others are taken by the Iranian and Iraqi women, who are having an argument.' 'Betty,' I said, 'find another tree.' And she will tell you in fun about it too."

Dame Nita acknowledged that women wanted recognition for what they did, not just monetary or material rewards. They needed to become full partners in society – people in the fullest sense of the word. It was her view that the UN Decade for Women saw only a partial improvement in women's lot. Women were still the prime sufferers in countries that were impoverished.

Nineteen eighty-five was a year of many achievements for Dame Nita because, as well as everything else, one of the nation's papers, the *Bajan*, had named her the West Indian of the Year. She was described as being "Strong as an ox, yet mild as a dove", a powerful manager who had all the combative spirit of a freedom fighter.[27]

Ambassador to the United Nations

When the UN General Assembly opened its session in mid September 1986, Dame Nita Barrow was one of the three women ambassadors of the 159 permanent representatives of their countries. Always a diplomat by nature and intuition, she was now officially appointed as such, Barbadian ambassador to the UN. This necessitated her moving on a more permanent basis to New York from her 'retired' domicile, Barbados. Dame Nita and Michele Landsberg, a well-known women's activist and journalist (whose husband Stephen Lewis was Canada's ambassador to the UN at the same time), were instantly drawn to each other by a shared political and feminist viewpoint, and by a common amusing title: ambassador extraordinary and plenipotentiary and permanent representative. Landsberg pointed out that, ironically, given Dame Nita's

> quiet and lifelong crusade against the waste and cruelty of prejudice, Dame Nita was prevented from reaching the career pinnacle she deserved by the twin idiocies of sexism and hierarchy. She was hotly touted for the presidency of the UN General Assembly during her term as ambassador; in that role, she might have deployed her shrewd communicating skills, efficiency and quick intelligence to propel forward the work of the United Nations. Instead, the job went to some ineffectual, now-forgotten but higher-ranking male nonentity.[28]

Dr Potter, too, remarked that "she brought to everything she did in the United Nations all the skills and experiences, which she had acquired on all the issues of our disturbed world. Indeed, it is said of her that she was the most respected and appreciated president that the United Nations General Assembly never had!"

Landsberg penned her fond remembrance of Dame Nita. It is, as so many other stories have been, connected with her cuisine. Dame Nita broke the mould of diplomatic dinners at her ambassador's home where her dinner parties were renowned for their ease, laughter and liveliness. "Surely, she was the only Ambassador Plenipotentiary who ever cooked and served her own curries. Later, when she came to Toronto on high-level visits, friends and acquaintances flocked to greet her in her hotel suite – a Nita sojourn was like a royal levee, with never fewer than a couple of dozen relatives and close friends crowding in, all to be introduced to strangers in the glow of Nita's generous praise."[29] Helen Mussallem shared a similar story, that "she taught me how to cook . . . I tried to watch her – you just watch, and then she told me after, 'You use your imagination and use a recipe as a guide' and she was excellent – the only head of state who did her own cooking!"

In 1987 yet another award was to come her way from the Caribbean: the Caribbean Community's Women's Award for her personal accomplishments and the stature she gave to the women of the Caribbean. A year later, she was the recipient of CARICOM's Triennial Award for her outstanding contribution to the development of women. It was also Nita's leadership style in the role and development of women that was commented on frequently. Dr Karen Sealey, Caribbean programme coordinator, PAHO/WHO, remarked:

> It has been a rare experience and one that I shall treasure for all my life – to have had the opportunity to work with someone as esteemed as Dame Nita in the field of public health. At a time when the organization and myself were on the footing of trying to expand what was happening in the Caribbean, Dame Nita's subtle guidance to make one not even realize when the guidance in fact was coming from the outside and not the inside was a characteristic that is rare in most human beings . . . Dame Nita encouraged her colleagues at PAHO to consider those who had not even in fact come unto the pages or been considered for attention . . . [30]

Carmen Lusan, her very close friend, also commented that "she was very good at listening. She asked questions if it were not very clear, to make sure that she understood what I was saying. She would try to find out what other people thought before we got her thoughts. She was an excellent person in the chair. That is why she got on so many committees." A listener, a clarifier, a peacemaker, a conciliator, an organizer, a negotiator, a quiet but firm advocate of the impoverished and the underprivileged. The story is told that at the 1985 UN Decade for Women Conference in Nairobi, Nita had reserved the front seats of this enormous gathering for the poor, rural women who were coming from the Kenyan villages, most of them having their first exposure to an event like this. She wanted to ensure that these unsophisticated women would be made to feel comfortable, as seats were at a premium due to the huge unexpected attendance. The press from around the world occupied the front seats to gain a good vantage point. Nita informed them that those seats had been reserved for the delegates, the women who had come from all the villages in Africa and that they were the ones for which the meeting was intended. The press initially refused to move but eventually did so as Nita in her quiet, firm manner said, "We are not going to start this meeting. You are press people and cannot take up the most important seats here."

Carmeta Fraser, Barbadian delegate to the UN women's conference in Copenhagen, was almost moved to tears when she paid her tribute to Dame Nita on her death in 1995. In a voice full of emotion, she shared her sentiments, simply and powerfully. She summed up all that Dame Nita truly was and the legacy for women in particular that she left behind:

On the home front, Dame Nita always wanted to have organizations that were strong, vibrant and who cared for the women out there – the women in agriculture, the women who were deprived, the women who had no husbands, the women who had lots of children and had serious problems. She was a person who was a very personal person to you. Up to last Sunday night she called me and ensured, before my birthday was over, to wish me a happy birthday. It is very unlikely that you get a person in such a high office interacting at the village level with people. To be interested in promoting local yam, local food all over the world, so that Barbados import food bills could come down – and indeed that was one of her dreams. Again, to see Nelson Mandela free was another dream that came true. Dame Nita had several dreams for the world, not just for Barbados. She has been a great inspiration to me. She has also been a source of comfort and people may not realize that she believed in not being religious but being Christian. She was the Christian in all her expressions and in her conduct. Because she would rather see a Christian than to hear about a Christian. In everything she went about to do she put God in front. Whenever she was asked to take on a post, even that of governor general, she said, 'I would have to pray about it first.' And that part of her inspired me even more . . . We are going to miss her sadly, but those of us who have been associated have been able to learn from her, and indeed she has always expressed to me her wish to see us continue and to keep the torch burning even although she might be long gone. She has always said that. And the greatest tribute I think I could pay to her is by God's help and grace to continue to fight and struggle to make Barbados a better and happier place for all of us to live. I can see her looking down from her eternal place in heaven because inasmuch as she has given it to one of the least and has done it to one of the least of the apostles and she has done it unto me and to all Barbadians, and to peoples of the world . . . The Bible says 'Rejoice again! I say Rejoice!', because the torch is there standing like a beacon, a woman who has given, a real daughter of the soil. She was a strict guardian of our heritage and indeed a firm craftsman of her faith . . . she lived for others and her living was not in vain.[31]

Never losing touch with her profession, always acknowledging her foundation in nursing, no matter how high in social status she moved, Dame Nita remained true to her roots – the Caribbean, women and nursing. The International Council of Nurses (ICN) in Korea honoured her in 1989 with the Christiane Reimann Award, often dubbed the 'Nobel Prize for Nursing'. It was only the second time that it had been offered in the history of nursing. The first winner, in 1985, was Virginia Henderson of the United States, a household name in the annals of nursing history. Always modest, Dame Nita's first reaction, on hearing that she was the winner of the award, was "absolute amazement". No one, however, in nursing and the health field was surprised. She was also the keynote speaker at that nineteenth quadrennial congress of nurses and, although she was ambassador to the UN from Barbados at the time, she had kept well abreast of the major issues facing nursing. Dame Nita skilfully used the watchword for the next quadrennium given by the outgoing president of the ICN, 'justice', as a springboard for her address and noted that while justice encompassed many facets of life there was none more than health care where so many injustices still prevailed. She reiterated her constant theme for accountability and primary health care and the role of nurses within these contexts in the global arena. Community care, forging partnerships with other disciplines and compassion were desperately needed and were some of the challenges facing nursing in the changing state of the world.[32]

Governor General

In November 1980 Queen Elizabeth II made Nita a Dame of the Order of St Andrew and St George, for extraordinary and outstanding achievement and merit in service to Barbados and humanity at large, on the recommendation of the prime minister of Barbados. Universities in the Caribbean, Canada and the United States have awarded her honorary degrees. Nita said that the two honours she held dearest to her heart were the one from her own people, UWI, and the other from McMaster University, Canada, as it was the first university to bestow on her an international honorary degree of Doctor of Sciences, in May 1982.

In retrospect, a final accolade to Nita's many achievements was the appointment as governor general of Barbados in 1990. Sadly, our interviews that would have covered her years as governor general never took place, so this section must instead conclude with some of the many tributes to Dame Nita when she died.

As governor general of Barbados, Dame Nita, the first woman in that role, was affectionately and appropriately called "the people's GG". She brought a natural dignity to that highest office and was deemed capable in her quiet manner of quelling the greatest storm and putting the most uncomfortable person at ease. Dame Nita received many tributes from around the world, and as Peter Morgan, former high commissioner for Barbados to Canada, so aptly said in his personal tribute to her at her funeral:

And so it is that during the next few days, you will read in the press and you will hear on the radio and television, tributes from around the world will come. These are routinely sent, government to government, when presidents, prime ministers, kings and queens and dignitaries pass away. But I want you to know that the vast majority of the tributes that will be sent on

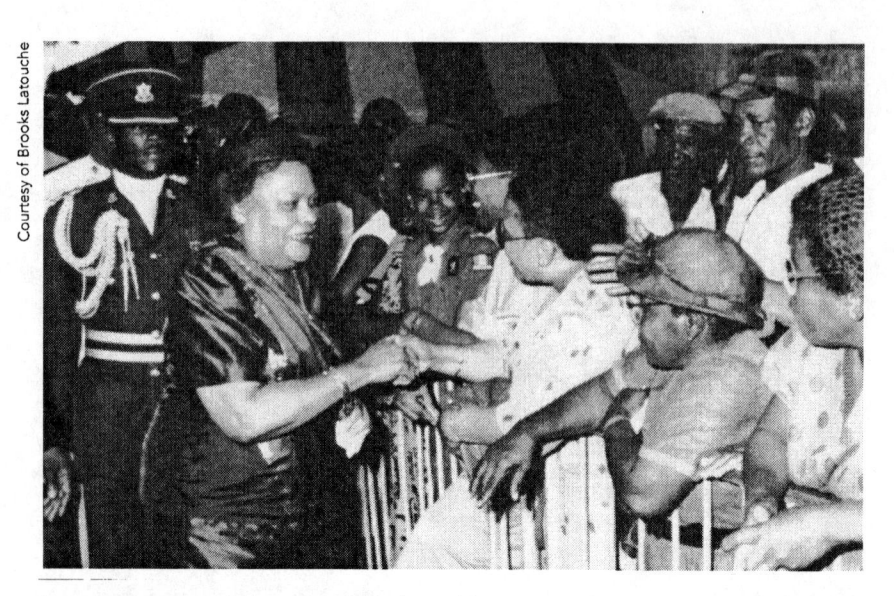

Dame Nita mixing with the crowds, Barbados, 1995

behalf of Dame Nita will be sent sincerely out of the affection and respect and the love which all of these people had for this lady. She will be greatly missed.[33]

He cited a few personal experiences to illustrate the great regard in which she was held by leaders around the world. One of the many he referred to was the Heads of Government Commonwealth Conference in Vancouver in 1987, which he and Dame Nita attended as part of the Barbadian delegation. The focus of attention at that Commonwealth Conference was the prime minister of India, Rajiv Gandhi, who was having trouble with the Sikh community and there was a big Sikh community in Vancouver making threats on his life. Morgan said,

There he was in the middle of the room, surrounded by all these press people, and suddenly across the room, he spotted Dame Nita. He pushed everybody aside and he strode across the room, flung open his arms, and said, 'Nita! Nita! How great to see you!' and they had a big embrace and I got introduced! It was like that all the way through the conference, she seemed to know everybody.[34]

Her many testimonials were in fact a series of anecdotal events of people's encounters with her. These were, of course, people who represented various organizations but there was no doubt that countless others were shared by the simple, everyday folk in Barbados, the Caribbean and globally. The Anglican bishop, Dr Rufus Brome, offered his story: "Who could not be touched by her personal notes written in her own handwriting. I treasure her letters of congratulation on the first anniversary of my ordination and consecration as a bishop and on the recent conferment of the degree of Doctor of Divinity." Such personal, human touches were what endeared her so much to all.

Peggy Antrobus, women's rights activist, Development Alternatives for Women (DAWN), gave one or two of her 'Nita stories':

Only today, for instance, when I was talking to somebody at one of the furniture manufacturers, and they were talking about having made some furniture for her and that they had never met her but they encountered her as a very kind voice. She called to thank them and this person said to me, 'You know, she could have asked her secretary to do it but she did it herself.' That is so typical of Dame Nita. I remember a story that I heard a couple of years ago, even when she was governor general. A woman called her, out of the blue, to say that her mother was dying and that her mother really wanted to meet Dame Nita. Dame Nita went to meet this woman so that she could give her that gift . . . Last year, when I hosted a meeting of the Network of Third World Women involved in promoting development alternatives (DAWN), Dame Nita made her beach house available to us so that we could have one day of our meeting away from the hotel. It was very important because she realized that we were stuck in the hotel for a series of back-to-back meetings planned over ten days. She thought that if we could have one day of our meeting in a different setting, it would combine – you know these women were from Africa, Asia, and the Southern Pacific – the opportunity of seeing another side of Barbados. That kind of consideration she showed for other people, I found very endearing . . . I remember in September, I wasn't able to go to the conference in Beijing, and she was invited as a keynote speaker for the opening of the forum and she couldn't go either. She invited me to Government House on the morning when the conference would have started, just so that we could spend some time talking a little bit about what was happening in Beijing. She was that kind of person.[35]

Dr Philip Potter, one of her dearest and oldest friends, in his homily at the state funeral in December 1995, observed that apart from her work in community health care, which was

the greatest of the many contributions she had made, . . . Nita's other abiding contribution was in the cause of women. She had no doubt in her mind, from her youth, that women were made like men in the image and likeness of God, and that our calling was to be a worldwide communion and community of women and men together in church and society. Nita carried this concern in a characteristic way. Not aggressive or excessive but by being herself commanding respect and demanding respect and space to live for her sisters all over the world. I would also say that she approached this very difficult, age-old problem in a Caribbean, calypso style . . . Nita helped women to equip themselves to have their own identity, their integrity in equality with men. And she did this by her own shining example . . . Her strength was to encourage women to take on the whole world agenda by preparing themselves to work for human rights, dignity, justice and peace for all.[36]

Dame Nita was given a state funeral befitting a person of her stature. It took place on 20 December 1995 from Government House to the St James Methodist Church and then for a private burial with relatives and close friends. This did not prevent the ordinary folk, however, from crowding around at the cemetery to witness, albeit at a distance, the final resting place of their beloved "people's GG".

Dame Nita Barrow, an unforgettable Caribbean nurse, who Blackman in his testimonial affirmed, "above all remains for all women and I hope for many men as well, an example of service with love and how to hold a continuing love affair with humanity".[37]

The year 1997 marked the fiftieth anniversary of the founding of the NAJ. On 20 March 1997 the association held a ceremony to unveil a bust in memory of Dame Nita, their first president. The bust is mounted in the lobby of the Mary Seacole Annexe of the headquarters of the NAJ. The event was chaired by the current president Pearlie Esteen with the unveiling of the bust by Grace March, the past president after Dame Nita. The citation was read by Syringa Marshall-Burnett, the current director of the Department of Advanced Nursing Education, and the guest speaker was Lady Standard, a nurse and close friend of Dame Nita, who resides in Jamaica. Some highlights of her remarks of their early days in training in 1940, when Dame Nita was a senior nurse and Lady Standard, a junior, was assigned to work with her on night duty, seemed appropriate to close this chapter on a truly gracious and rare woman. Lady Standard's words echo, then as now, the salient characteristics of Dame Nita:

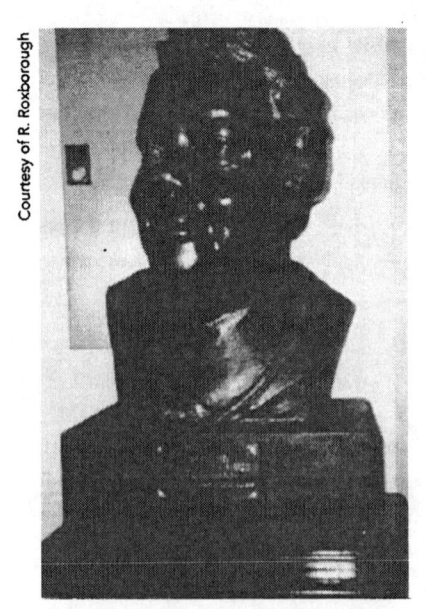

Bust of Dame Nita in the Nurses' Association of Jamaica lobby, Kingston, Jamaica

Nurse Barrow was one of those Seniors who spared no effort in caring for her patients, and she expected the same from everyone who worked with her. To her co-workers, she was always kind, considerate and caring, sharing her knowledge along the way, so that at the end of my two months night duty with her, I began to feel like a real nurse.[38]

Dame Nita Barrow, governor general of Barbados, born in a small West Indian island, always acknowledged her debt to her many relatives and others who guided her in her growth towards her pinnacle of achievement but, most of all, she saw that honour as a tribute to the many sacrifices of Barbadian women. She was, and will remain forever, a beacon of light for Caribbean nurses and women throughout the world.

Notes

1. Ann Jacobs, personal interview, December 1995. All material quoted from Jacobs is from this interview.
2. Mavis Harney, personal interview, December 1995. All material quoted from Harney is from this interview.
3. C. Sunshine, *The Caribbean-Survival, Struggle and Sovereignty,* Part I. Ecumenical Program for Interamerican Communication and Action (EPICA) (Washington, DC: EPICA, 1973), 2–45.
4. The study that Nita referred to was the subject of Helen Mussallem's doctoral thesis, "Spotlight on Nursing Education: A Report of the Pilot Project for the Evaluation of Schools of Nursing in Canada", which examined the standards of nursing education in the diploma schools of nursing in Canada
5. Helen Mussallem, telephone interview, May 1997. All material quoted from Mussallem is from this interview.
6. Federal Government of the West Indies, Barbados, Report of Conference of Nursing Administrators, Bridgetown, Barbados, 31 August–6 September 1959, Appendix V, 1.
7. Ibid., Res. 182.
8. PAHO/WHO, *Survey of Schools of Nursing in the Caribbean Area,* Reports on Nursing, no. 6 (Washington, DC: PAHO/WHO, 1966), 16.
9. This referred to the Canadian survey done by Helen; the Château Laurier is a luxurious hotel in Ottawa.
10. PAHO/WHO, *Survey of Schools,* 73–77.

11. PAHO/WHO, *Resurvey of Schools of Nursing in the Caribbean Area*, Reports on Nursing, no. 15, vol. 1, Nursing Education (Washington, DC: PAHO/WHO, 1971). See also E.K. Walters, *Nursing: A History from the Late Eighteenth–Late Twentieth Century Barbados* (Bridgetown, Barbados: E.K. Walters, 1995), chapter 13 in particular; Government of Trinidad and Tobago, Ministry of Health, Report of First Conference of Caribbean Health Ministers, 11–14 February 1969.
12. Carmen Lusan, telephone interview, June 1997. All material quoted from Lusan is from this interview.
13. CMC/WCC, "CMC Study/Enquiry: The Roots", *Contact* 51 (June 1979): 1, 11.
14. Ibid.
15. See F.W. Blackman, *Dame Nita: Caribbean Woman, World Citizen* (Kingston, Jamaica: Ian Randle Publishers, 1995), chapter 4, 65–89, for a full exposition of Nita's involvement with the CMC.
16. C. Barnard, "Dame Nita Barrow: An Outstanding Woman", *Bajan,* January/February 1986, 19.
17. Ibid.
18. Dr Potter, eulogy, *Dame Nita Barrow's Funeral* (Barbados Information Services, videotape, 20 December 1995).
19. CMC/WCC, "The Annual Meeting of the Christian Medical Commission", *Contact* 39 (April 1977): 3.
20. N. Barrow, "Nursing: The Art, Science and Vocation in Evolution", *Contact* 59 (December 1980): 1–13, 18.
21. Ibid.
22. R. Kidd, *Whilst Time Is Burning: A Report on Education for Development* (Ottawa: International Development Research Centre, 1974).
23. In 1958 Roby Kidd conducted an enquiry in the Caribbean funded by the Carnegie Corporation and supported by the UCWI. See Nancy Cochrane et al., *J.R. Kidd: An International Legacy of Learning* (Vancouver: Centre for Continuing Education, 1986), for a detailed account of Roby's work, especially chapter 6 which deals with the Caribbean.
24. See Blackman, *Dame Nita,* chapter 6, for a more detailed rendition of Nita's involvement with the ICAE.
25. Sir Shridath Ramphal, tribute to Dame Nita, *Dame Nita Barrow's Funeral* (Barbados Information Services, videotape, 20 December 1995).
26. N. Barrow, "The Role of Women in International Development" (Address given at the University of Alberta, Edmonton, Alberta, 10 March 1987).
27. Ibid.; Barnard, "Dame Nita Barrow".
28. M. Landsberg, "World Says Goodbye to One Grand Dame", *Toronto Star,* 23 December 1995.

29. Ibid.
30. Karen Sealey, tribute, *Dame Nita Barrow's Funeral* (Barbados Information Services, videotape, 20 December 1995).
31. Carmeta Fraser, tribute, *Dame Nita Barrow's Funeral* (Barbados Information Services, videotape, 20 December 1995).
32. N. Barrow, "Nursing: A New Tomorrow", *International Nursing Review* 36, no. 5 (1989): 141–44.
33. Peter Morgan, tribute, *Dame Nita Barrow's Funeral* (Barbados Information Services, videotape, 20 December 1995).
34. Ibid.
35. Peggy Antrobus, tribute, *Dame Nita Barrow's Funeral* (Barbados Information Services, videotape, 20 December 1995).
36. Phillip Potter, tribute, *Dame Nita Barrow's Funeral* (Barbados Information Services, videotape, 20 December 1995).
37. 'Woodie' Blackman, tribute, *Dame Nita Barrow's Funeral* (Barbados Information Services, videotape, 20 December 1995).
38. Evelyn Standard, "Dame Nita Barrow" (paper presented at the unveiling of a bust in memory of Dame Nita Barrow by the Nurses' Association of Jamaica, 20 March 1997, Mona, Jamaica).

PART II
Berenice Dolly

When a woman tells the truth she is creating the possibility for more truth around her.

Adrienne Rich

Courtesy of Ben Dolly

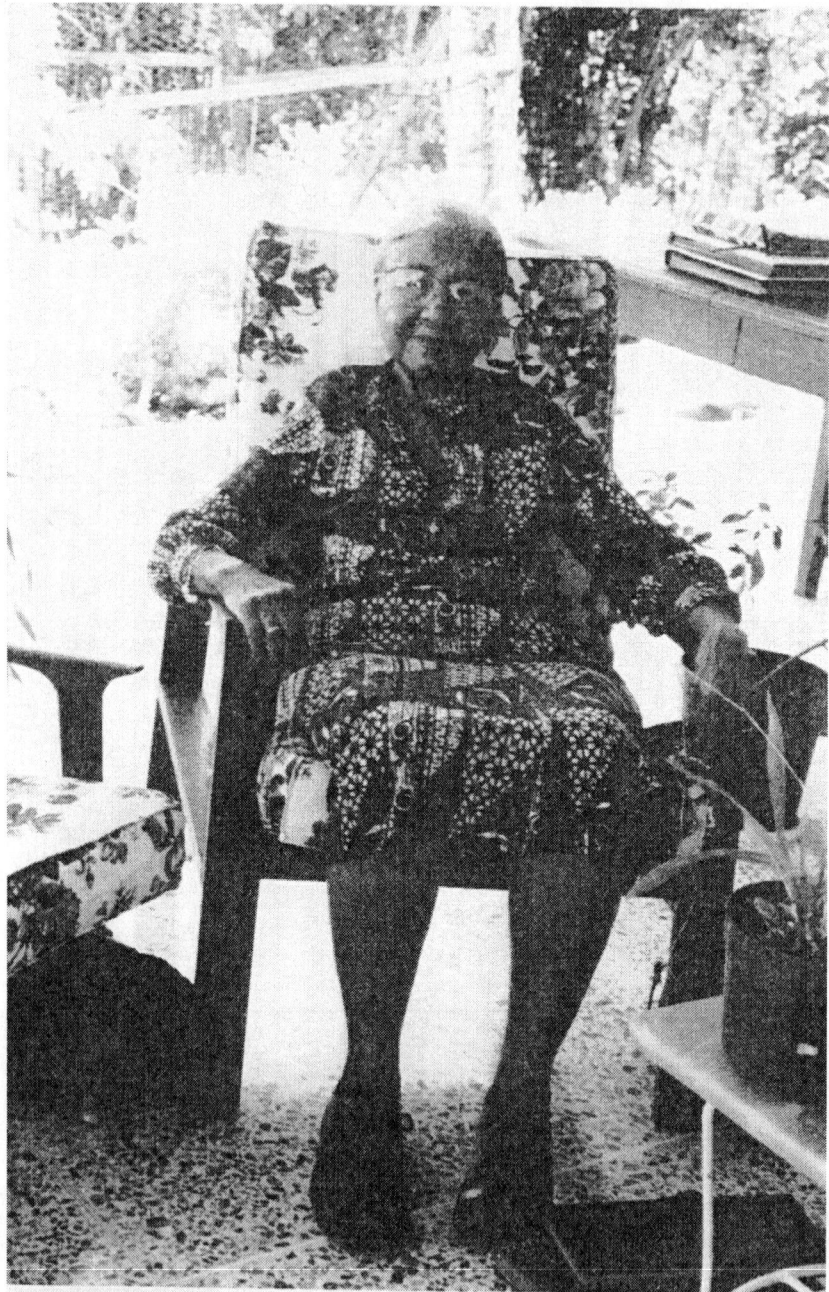

Ben Dolly, Pointe-à-Pierre, Trinidad, 1996

Chapter Three

A Woman of Action

On a warm tropical night in 1996, I arrived by car at the Pointe-à-Pierre compound of Petrotrin, the site of the oil refineries of Trinidad and Tobago. As I waited at the entrance by the guard booth, I soon saw, or barely saw, a tiny grey-haired lady wearing spectacles, driving towards us in a rather battered-looking Mazda 323, 1982 model. Her hair was pulled tightly back in a bun, with a scarf supporting it. Berenice Dolly greeted us warmly and I transferred to her car for what would be two intensive and enjoyable days of interviews and discoveries.

The following morning in brilliant sunshine, as we sat on the family's porch, surrounded by several pots of orchids, her favourite plant and hobby, Berenice Dolly (affectionately known everywhere as Ben) described some of the highlights of her professional life. We spent some time talking about her love of orchids and her care of them, then she took me to see one of her colleagues. Driving with Ben is an experience; she is rather like a Miss Marple, seemingly oblivious of the traffic, yet arriving safe and sound to our destination. Her repeated admonition to me was, "You don't trust me!" as I clung tightly to the door. I do not recall seeing seat belts. I must confess that I was frightened the entire trip.

Her small stature belied a compelling character. At seventy-nine, Ben continued to be a woman of action. The phone never ceased ringing, and yet Ben was able to coordinate numerous activities while being interviewed. For example, while I was there one morning, the manager of her estate paid a visit to discuss business matters, cocoa beans were spread on the ground drying, the gardeners arrived to tend the lawn, the housekeeper arrived for cleaning. Her husband, Dr Reynold Dolly, was ill and confined to his bedroom so Ben served him his meals. Hilary, her youngest daughter who lives with them, was also ill and Ben checked in on her, then she drove me to the club on the compound to fetch our lunch, and so it went on. In the midst of all this she found time to water her orchids.

Ben is an avid orchid horticulturist and her home is full of trophies won in a variety of exhibitions. She has been a member of the Trinidad Orchid Society since 1961, participating actively in horticultural shows. Her daughter Joan has an orchid garden and Ben proudly told me that her grandson Adrian is now a judge in the Orchid Society and that from time to time, when he was a little boy, he would accompany her to orchid meetings and call himself 'the orchid man'.

Another of her pastimes is playing bridge which for Ben "is a wonderful, intellectual exercise that everyone should indulge in. No matter what age, sex or nationality, if you can find someone who can sit at a table, you can have a useful occupation." Those are her two major loves – her orchids and playing bridge – amidst all her professional and community endeavours.

Ben Grant and Reynold Dolly were married in 1940 shortly after Ben graduated from basic training as a nurse. She opined, "I really felt at that point in time that it meant an end to my nursing career." Although she expected she would have to leave nursing to devote herself to her family responsibilities, she soon found outlets for her energy and natural leadership. There was the opportunity to continue in nursing affairs through involvement in her professional organization, and seize it she did. Ben, by nature, is not 'laid back'. Assertive and constantly seeking challenges for personal and professional growth, she continued to develop herself and utilize her many talents. She quickly got involved with the Ministry of Health in San Fernando and a host of voluntary organizations including the Chest and Heart Association and the Coterie of Social Workers, founded by Audrey Jeffers, to which she made a lifelong contribution. In San Fernando she worked in nursery schools for the Coterie. Always sharp and shrewd, Ben was involved in activities which would make use of her background and expertise and also enable her to continue developing both within and beyond nursing. She was fortunate in that her professional organization held annual 'updates', which gave nurses who were not actually at the bedside in the hospital the opportunity to serve in some capacity.

Dr Dolly had worked in the government service for seven years and then, in 1943, took up a post as a junior medical officer at Pointe-à-Pierre Hospital in the south of the island where the oil refineries are located. The hospital is a private institution built by the oil companies, mainly to serve the personnel of the industry and its surroundings. The refineries are contained within a guarded compound where local persons and foreigners are employed in a variety of professional, technical and clerical positions. Homes are provided for key professionals in the residential area. The oil company when the Dollys arrived was originally British Oil, and late in the colonial period it was taken over by Texaco. Today it is a national industry run by the Government of Trinidad and Tobago under the name Petrotrin.

The Dollys have lived there ever since their arrival in 1943. The noteworthiness of this and Dr Dolly's subsequent rise to senior positions for him, a black man, albeit a physician, within the oil industry on that compound, warrants some discussion of the nation's historical past, as his position and location had a significant bearing on Ben's life and contributions.

REMEMBERING THE PAST

Trinidad and Tobago, discovered by Columbus in 1498, are two islands in the southernmost part of the Caribbean Sea that constitute an independent unitary state. The island of Tobago lies about twenty-six miles northeast of Trinidad and was essentially a sugar colony. To provide additional labour for the plantations, after emancipation in 1834, the British introduced East Indian immigrants as indentured labour from 1845 to 1917.[1] In 1899 the island was amalgamated with Trinidad to form one colony while retaining its own legal and fiscal systems.

The population of the twin islands, estimated at 1,272,385 as of July 1996, consists of about 40 percent blacks, 40 percent East Indians, with the remainder being of European, Chinese or mixed descent; the combinations are numerous. Trinidad's religious diversity is even more bewildering than its racial complexity. Roman Catholics constitute 33.6 percent, Hindus 25 percent, Anglicans 15 percent, Muslims 5.9 percent, Presbyterians 3.9 percent and a host of other

Christian and non-Christian sects the remaining 16.6 percent. Class distinction is common to all the major racial and religious categories. Trinidad has basically a class structure, with multiracial and multicultural groupings in each of the three hierarchical strata.[2]

Three decisive events took place in Trinidad in the first half of the twentieth century that changed the history of the island. The first was the discovery of oil in commercial quantities in 1910. The second was the abolition by the indentured system of Indian labour in 1917, based in large part on opposition of the nationalist movement in India. The third was the emergence of the working class movement, after World War I, led by a radical European planter of Corsican extraction, Captain Arthur Cipriani. He was in close communication with the British Labour Party and formed the socialist Trinidad Labour Party.[3]

In both the sugar and oil industries, located in the southern part of the island, there was an explosive social situation arising out of the discontent of workers, blacks and Indians, who had no legitimate means of expressing their grievances. In the late 1930s, widespread violence erupted, originating with the oilfield workers led by a Uriah Butler, a black man originally from Grenada, and an emotional mass leader. While Butler was never able to mobilize mass support, he and his colleagues precipitated the rise of trade unions that proceeded to become independent forces of their own. They engineered the direct entry of the working class into colonial politics.[4]

The Moyne Commission visited Trinidad and Tobago as it did Barbados and Jamaica and for the same reason: to investigate the local social, economic and political situation. In dealing with Trinidad and Tobago in its report of 1938, the commission pointed out the need to address public health concerns, and called for the appointment of indigenous physicians to leadership roles in the hospitals. The commission also found that sugar production in Trinidad and Tobago had doubled in ten years, and that Trinidad had become the leading producer of oil in the empire, accounting for 62.8 percent of production in 1936. Concurrent with this economic picture was the deplorable economic and social conditions of the workers. The Indian population in particular was riddled with hookworm. Malaria and hookworm were the leading causes of death and debility in workers, a result of the unsanitary conditions which existed on the agricultural estates and the surrounding villages. Recommendations for improvement were made but little could be achieved until the end of World War II in 1945.

The postwar years saw the introduction of full adult franchise in 1946 and the first elections held under universal suffrage, the maturation of the trade union movement, and the intensification of the movement for self-government and federation. By 1955 the first genuinely successful mass nationalist movement appeared on the scene, which culminated in independence in 1962, thus ending British colonialism. In 1976 Trinidad and Tobago became an independent republic governed by its own president instead of the British monarch.

Not the Usual Housewife

The social and political climate in the 1940s was ripe for the entry of blacks into leadership positions, positions previously occupied by whites only. The health field was a perfect choice for introducing such a policy of integration, considering the call of the Moyne Commission for the advancement of local physicians. It could have influenced management in the oil industry to consider appointing qualified blacks to key positions, and a logical step in that direction would be in the field of health care.

Reynold (Rey) Dolly was the first black physician to be appointed junior medical officer at the Pointe-à-Pierre Hospital. He remained there as a salaried physician and never went into private practice. Over the years he rose to be chief medical officer, then director of the medical services for the whole company and, finally, a director of Texaco. Although he retired some time ago, he was retained as a consultant and the Dollys have remained in their home on the compound. This beautiful setting, surrounded by a variety of tropical trees, myriad exotic shrubs and flowering plants is the background from which Ben carried and still carries out her manifold activities.

Ben was loth to accept being considered a woman of means. It was her contention that Rey had worked hard for whatever they had achieved financially. However, she conceded, "We were in a specially privileged position in that many services were laid on which you could not have been able to get elsewhere." The location and her close association with the hospital where her husband worked allowed her to have access to many friends and colleagues who, like herself, lived on the compound. Many had the time available to assist her and she expressed gratitude to them for giving their expertise and skill to many causes on the island whenever she called upon them. Some were nurses who had worked and trained abroad and were happy to be of assistance.

Ben talked about Rey and his contribution to her development. She believed in a man being the head of the household as long as it was understood that each person must be allowed to develop. And develop they both did. While it is generally accepted in the island that the husband is the head of the household and therefore determines where the family lives, it is most unusual for someone of her age to hold such a radical viewpoint. Dr Dolly was completely absorbed in his profession and his sports – he was a great athlete. She gave him credit, saying, "He did not put any restrictions on either my time or what money I spent, which was money that he worked for and it was very small, may I tell you . . . His contribution is that he put no barriers at all to my time or using his means or using the opportunities that he had. He allowed me to use all these things without hesitation." Despite her gratitude to Rey and not gainsaying his supportiveness, well into the twentieth century, 'respectable' women of all races in the Caribbean did not enter the workplace but engaged in home activities and 'good works', pioneering activities of all types but especially those concerned with women.[5] Ben Dolly was such a prototype.

While Dr Dolly was not wealthy, the family was privileged as there were opportunities that were afforded him and, consequently, Ben and their children which many others did not have at that time. They had access to a telephone when many did not; they enjoyed paid leave every three years when they travelled to England. However, Ben said, "It was not always money that enabled you to help people. I find that . . . one of the blessings of being in the health field is knowing what to do or knowing where to go to get something done . . . Money was not considered at all. People worked and enjoyed their work regardless of what they got." The fact that Ben used those opportunities to help others is what characterized her and made her an outstanding role model of her time. Arguably, Ben and Rey were not your usual married couple of that period. Ben allowed that the world has changed, and that it was also the fact that in the midst of all these activities, she had good domestic help. She had a housekeeper who had been in her family since Ben was born and who lived with them as a permanent member of the family. Besides that, there were other people who helped with the children, allowing her the freedom to do volunteer work.

However, although many middle class families could afford domestic help, not all women felt motivated to volunteer their services as freely as Ben did. Religion and social work were the only legitimate areas of activity for women who chose to contribute outside of the home. And this Ben did with much gusto. She epitomized the middle class educated 'lady' of her day. Social work could convey much honour and prestige on the men and women of their class. Moreover, encompassed within the concept of social work was the quality of selflessness. This apparent selflessness

A Woman of Action

in women – concern for others – was one of the pillars of the Western European ideology which Ben represented. This imported Western model was the model for 'correct' behaviour for women.[6] Ben was among those few activist women in her commitment to serve society. It was her belief that if an opportunity for service presented itself, then it was intended to be used and that it took little effort to do so. She bemoaned the fact that nursing and all professions were getting more specialized with experts in one area having a less broad, general knowledge base. It was because of her broad-based knowledge that she was able to help others in need. Her deep faith and convictions came forth as she elaborated, "I honestly believe that if you take time or knowledge or whatever to serve somebody else, the good Lord will look after your needs. You don't have to worry about it. Leave it to Him. Trust Him . . . He places these opportunities before you, for you to benefit from it and use it for somebody. Otherwise, what is the sense in hoarding it up? . . . I have had so much exposure that I did not seek, it just came my way that I feel that I need to pass it on." Her attempt to improve the prestige and status of black and coloured middle-class women in the eyes of society were carried out through her active participation in social work, in black women's organizations and activities, in nursing, and in the colonial political structure.

An active member of the Roman Catholic church, Ben was very involved in church work. She and Rey were involved in study groups. She is a woman of deep faith and credited this strong belief to her mother who was a woman who "lived by faith. She believed and trusted God and so I grew up knowing that, and I can easily accept whatever comes, good or bad and know very well it was God's will . . . It has been a great comfort to me at all times." Also, Ben as a young girl was a member of the Legion of Mary, a young women's religious group. As a student nurse, she formed a unit, a Praesidium, in the hospital, which met at two different times to accommodate students and nurses on day and night shifts. This was a revolutionary idea in the church and permission had to be granted from Ireland. The mission of the group is concerned with Catholic education, counselling and other spiritual endeavours.

In her later years, Ben was on the parish council and was always willing to lend a hand whenever needed. She mused, "I think this saying that busy people always find time to do things is true. Because you're in action. And while you are doing one thing, you have the opportunity to do something else, without any effort."

Ben's Family

None of Ben and Rey's children – Joan, Stephen or Hilary – followed in their parent's field. Ben expressed some disappointment at this as she had wanted at least one to be in a health profession. When they were growing up they would say to their parents, "I know what I'm not going to be. I'm not going to be a doctor or a nurse because you're never at home at night and you're working all the time." With much pride in her voice, she related the success of her children. The eldest, Joan Massiah, went into the diplomatic service. She served as a foreign officer and her most recent posting was in Washington as deputy ambassador. She is currently a permanent secretary in the Office of the Prime Minister in Port of Spain. She is married with one son, Adrian, who is the apple of his grandmother's eye. Lorna Rigsby, a friend of Ben for over fifty years, gave me an anecdote about Ben and Adrian when he was quite little. People were sometimes quite diffident in opposing Ben's point of view or querying her opinion. Adrian and his grandmother were playing a game but she did not understand some aspects of it, so he proceeded to correct her and 'put her in her place'. It was the first time that she had such a challenge to her authority and had to 'bow out', and Ben just loved it. She laughed while she recounted this story to Lorna, who added, "there was mutual respect".[7] Adrian recently graduated from the University of Pennsylvania and is doing postgraduate work in business.

Both Joan and Hilary, the youngest, went to UWI and majored in French, then spent a year at the Sorbonne in France. Hilary teaches French at St Joseph's Convent, a girls' secondary school in Port of Spain. It is ironic that sixty years or so later the very school her mother had declined to attend because of its predominantly white, privileged students was now the school where her daughter taught. From time to time, Hilary has travelled with students to Europe and she has received an award from the French government for promoting French culture. Stephen, born between two sisters, studied civil aviation in Scotland. He is a captain with the national airline, British West Indian Airways, and makes his home in Tobago.

Ben, somewhat defensive in talking about her children and her involvement in many community endeavours during their childhood, expressed her philosophy about sharing and rearing: "I do feel that children should grow up knowing that everything they have should be shared, including their parents. I don't think that persons who are all-absorbed with their children and do nothing else do anything to help those children . . . I think that children should know that they have a responsibility to the community in which they live. I hope I was right. I have no qualms letting them grow up and see that I felt it was my duty to share some of the gifts that God gave me, which I didn't do anything to deserve especially, with other people . . . They must have responsibility for the general good, apart from just what's happening in their own home. And I hope that it worked." This was Ben on her high moral ground, which she said her children called "preaching". It was her contention that "children have a full agenda when they start school and they never really come back to you again. Women who say they must stay at home want to feel indispensable." This coming from a woman born long before the word 'feminist' was in vogue. Although Ben would hardly characterize herself as a feminist, an activist she was and is, in a quiet yet determined way.

Joan Massiah, in retrospect, sees herself rather like her mother in many ways. "Strong, dominant, domineering" were some of the terms used. She described her mother as a very dominant personality who lived by 'the book' and one of the most remarkable people she had ever known. She continued, "She knows everything. I can call and ask her anything, from how many raisins to put in this to how many teaspoons of fertilizer to put on a plant or whatever. She's a storehouse of knowledge in every possible field. There isn't anything that you can ask her that she can't either give you the answer or tell you exactly where to go to find the answer."[8] She conceded, however, that growing up in Ben's household was not easy. On the one hand, she felt that her mother should have been at home more and, on the other, she rather enjoyed the freedom of "doing my own thing". This realization of how unusual was her mother's lifestyle was thrust upon her because all her friends' mothers were at home and they constantly drew her attention to the fact that her mother was not. The mother of one of her friends said, "Hi Joan, where is your mother this morning? What time did she go out this morning? I tried to get her at half-past six and she seemed to be out already." Such encounters made Joan feel guilty. As she expressed it, "I don't think that it was something that if we had been left on our own we would necessarily have come to that conclusion ourselves, because we were always well taken care of, everything that was needed to be done was done, and I think as a mother myself, I suppose in later years I began to appreciate that . . . I didn't like it when people said to me 'Where is your mother? Why isn't she at home?' because it was an attack on her that I didn't like . . . I may have felt that she should have been there."

Gender-role stereotyping consistent with Victorian England expectations was clearly evident in these women where the woman's vocation was seen as that of wife and mother and whose true locus was the home. Joan was proud that her mother had a full life and afforded them the opportunity to be independent, encouraging them, yet without giving them free licence.

Stephen, Ben's only son, agreed with what his sister said about Ben; that she was strong-willed, principled and unafraid to express her opinions. He stressed that her absence from home did not harm them and that they were encouraged to be independent. He was fiercely protective about his mother: "Never did I feel she neglected me or we felt uncared for and unattended to . . . no matter what time of the night she came home . . . she would always come in to say goodnight and tell me what happened . . . There were times when she might come very late in the morning . . . but I never felt that it was neglect. We were allowed to do what we wanted within the boundaries of what a child is allowed to do. Always a strong character . . . Very old-fashioned in some ways, but progressive in so many others . . . Principled to a point and very inflexible in that area."[9]

Stephen's respect and high regard for his parents was shown by his assertions that while they were the only black family in Pointe-à-Pierre for many years, they were never made to feel that they were inferior. "We were taught to be the best you can be and we did." He showed great tenderness for his mother when he said, "She's a person who cares deeply for all of us and also for the things she puts her mind to. I think there are times when you want to be affectionate but you . . . unless you know her, you would not really know that there is this soft, caring, loving person behind the strengths that she has exhibited. She's a very warm and tender person, but she doesn't show her feelings." This restraint was also mentioned by Joan. The family did not have an open display of affection, except for Hilary who was very affectionate as a child, "hugging and kissing and it was always reciprocated".

They were brought up in a rather strict and prayerful home. In Stephen's words, "It was difficult to have a tiff because you were always told to be quiet. Well, you know you were out of place. So there could be no tiffs because there was no room for argument . . . There's nothing wrong with a family praying together and staying together, as the saying goes, but I personally feel that maybe too much was done."

Hilary was aware of the very busy life that her mother led when she was growing up. At times she resented it. Like her sister, her conflicting feelings were mirrored in her statements: "I think we were well taken care of, but not necessarily by her. My recollection of her was always on the go, always running in from one meeting and out to the next, for five minutes, and out . . . I used to get a bit angry because she always seemed to commit herself to everything, but yet there were family things that we did together. Quality time or dinner table or Sunday lunches or that sort

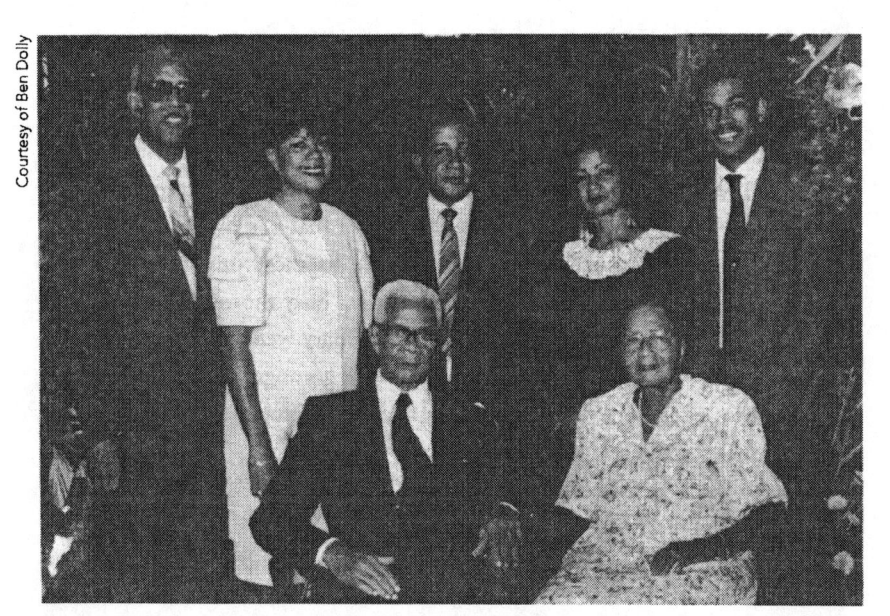

Ben and her family in Maraval, Trinidad, on her fiftieth wedding anniversary, 1996. Seated, Ben and her husband, Rey; standing, from left to right, Arthur Massiah (son-in-law), Joan Massiah (daughter), Stephen (son), Hilary (daughter), Adrian (grandson)

of thing. As I grew older, I think I then started to become aware of what she was really doing. As a child, maybe there was a little bit of a feeling that we wanted to see more of her. As I got older I started to understand the various things that she was involved in and started to appreciate that."[10]

Ben was regarded as a fountain of knowledge. Hilary's words confirmed those of Joan: "We are very independent, all of us. Independent, but dependent on her because she knows everything. She is a whiz brain with any problem you have. Anything you want to know in the world . . . how to make something in the kitchen, even though she's not a housewife . . . to how to address so and so letter, or what to put in it, or anything." Hilary described her mother as "a very wise and tremendous person. Wise to the point of intolerance. Very headstrong and is always right . . . Invariably she ended up being right which made things worse. Overpowering at times." She allowed that although they were very close they were all permitted their own space. She gently conceded that probably being the last she "felt stifled a bit . . . because she controlled me. She's that sort of person. Very, very controlling. Even now . . . she gets very frustrated because she cannot physically be as independent as she wants to be and has had to give in to us."

Hilary returned home to live with her parents in Pointe-à-Pierre, as they were ageing and Dr Dolly was not well (he died in 1999). She gave me an example of her mother's fiercely independent nature. Hilary had just returned home one afternoon and called out a greeting to her mother. The housekeeper said that Ben was out and would be back in five minutes. Eventually the housekeeper caved in and told Hilary that she was not supposed to tell her that Ben had gone to Port of Spain for a meeting. Port of Spain is a considerable distance from Pointe-à-Pierre, about an hour's drive in rather unsafe terrain and a busy thoroughfare, and Ben drove herself. The tables have turned indeed, as Hilary went on, "Even now she wants to do things because she knows we're going to get angry so she tries to sneak out. But she is unbelievably busy. Busy, busy and cannot stop. And when she stops, you know that something is wrong with her."

Ben has never admitted to having experienced racial discrimination overtly, yet it was an undercurrent in what her children said. Ben and Rey very carefully shielded their children from any racial problems. For instance, Joan's perception of racial discrimination was that the only problems were at home, because they were taught that, if there were a problem, they had to understand that they were different. She expanded, "I mean we couldn't run about barefoot and do the things that everybody else did because we were almost on trial. To some extent I resented that and I think as a girl it was more difficult for me than Stephen." Hilary speculated that when her parents first went to Pointe-à-Pierre that "She [Ben] herself, I think, suffered as a young wife and that I think was instrumental in her becoming so involved in her social activities to get out of there. She wasn't having coffee mornings . . . but as the years went by, I think they were very well accepted."

As a teenager, Hilary desperately wanted her parents to be more like the traditional couple who left home together to attend parties or events and returned home together. She said, "I always knew them going in opposite directions. Daddy going to his sports meeting and Mummy going to her Coterie, and if there was a party that they would be invited to, they would meet at the party from their respective meetings." But the Dollys never fitted a conventional mould. The fact that he was the first black physician to hold a medical post in the oilfields was in itself an unusual phenomenon and they were also the first black family to live on the compound. Dr Dolly not only had a busy practice but he was actively involved in cricket and other sports.

Hilary recalled their fiftieth wedding anniversary celebration to illustrate her point: "I remember the day . . . At the end of the mass I wanted them to walk down the aisle together. Typical, Mummy shot off to talk to the choir and Daddy somewhere else, and I just felt that that was symbolic to me of their whole relationship. She went this way, he went that way. And eventually . . . there is one picture of them coming down the aisle, but that is about three-quarters of the way down the church. But that symbolizes . . . I don't know if I ever said it to anybody, but that symbolizes their relationship to me. *Close but apart. Daddy gave Mummy her space*" (emphasis mine).

They exemplified what the famous Lebanese poet and philosopher, Kahlil Gibran, wrote on marriage in his acclaimed book *The Prophet*:

. . . But let there be spaces in your togetherness,
And let the winds of the heavens dance between you.
Love one another, but make not a bond of love:
. . . And stand together yet not too near together:
For the pillars of the temple stand apart,
And the oak tree and the cypress grow not in each other's shadow.[11]

Ben's friend from childhood, Lorna Rigsby, confirmed what the family acknowledged: that one of Ben's priorities was her family, and it was through their support that she was able to respond positively when called upon. Lorna's view was that Ben was strong and steadfast, and that while she possessed these qualities of strength and steadfastness, she was also a very cautious person who weighed all the pros and cons before embarking on any project. Lorna said, "She does not make judgments or decisions or statements without having thought about it . . . She's a woman of integrity, foresight and a leader. She's an achiever. She has a very positive attitude and she faces the hurdles that have to be overcome. She has the ability to put things in perspective." Lorna said of Ben, "She's been a dutiful daughter, she's been a wife, a mother, a grandmother, a nurse, a social and community worker, an agriculturist and much, much more . . . a multifaceted woman whose greatest asset is her keen sense of awareness. She's always aware of conditions and circumstances surrounding her. The environmental, social, economic, religious, or whatever . . . she realized that her career was in nursing, and not a career as any career, but as a vocation. And to this day, Ben is totally committed to this appreciation of nursing . . . Her friendship extends to anyone who is desperately in need of comfort, advice, solace in times of crisis. Ben is always there for them . . . She has done Trinidad and Tobago proud in her representation overseas at conferences and meetings, both with her professional status and her enormous contributions to community and social work at quality level . . . She's a very human person. I think this has been appreciated, by not only her friends and colleagues, but by the nation." This appreciation of her worth was indeed recognized as early as 1962 when she was made an Officer of the Most Excellent Order of the British Empire (OBE).

Women's Organizations

An interesting aspect of Ben's life is her participation in women's organizations. One that had influenced her as a schoolgirl would be with her all her life. It was the Coterie of Social Workers and was spearheaded by Audrey Jeffers, herself an extraordinary person. A formidable woman, she was one of the earliest role models for black women and a key person whose life and work influenced Ben. Audrey Jeffers was a highly educated woman of independent means who was one of the first black women to be elected to City Council in the early fifties. She had gone to Tranquillity Girls' Practising School for her primary and secondary education and then went to London and completed a diploma in social science. She became an eminent social worker and pioneer in voluntary social work in the island. While there were many people who did social work connected with their churches, it was Audrey Jeffers who brought it to public awareness in a profound way. Her entire life was dedicated to social service. In 1921 she founded the Coterie of Social Workers and its purpose was to feed schoolchildren, look after day nurseries, care for the blind, and address every conceivable type of social deprivation for the black underprivileged children and women in the island. But equally importantly, it unintentionally served as a vehicle for raising the status of black middle-class women (and men) in the society.[12]

When Ben was a teenager at Bishop Anstey High School, Audrey Jeffers' life and her movement, which was in its infancy, greatly influenced Ben. The Coterie gave young girls the opportunity to participate in events and functions, and to assist in community work. Ben was exposed to the Coterie at an early age and it heightened her sense of community contribution. Moreover, Mrs Pinheiro, with whom Ben boarded, was a member, so Ben attended all the functions which they organized to raise money for social causes. She read for the blind and, as a Girl Guide, would visit the elderly and the blind in their homes. Ben spoke with deep passion about this movement in the island during her youth and the significance of Audrey's impact: "She introduced you to work, to caring. You had to help. It was a general movement in the country, especially in Port of Spain and we were exposed to it. I was not conscious at the time of these things taking perhaps such a big part in my life. It just happened. That was the environment in which I grew. You had your school work to do . . . We were just drawn into it and the general awareness in the country at the time, of the need to help one another, to see that everybody was equipped to cope with the situation and gradually, I suppose, it was building up to nationhood . . . At all times, you had to know what was going on."

In 1947, when Ben was living in San Fernando, Audrey invited her to join the Coterie and to take over the chairmanship of the Day Nursery Committee. Ben remained on that committee for a number of years. Her role entailed fund raising, the maintenance of the buildings, staff salaries, feeding and caring for the children. Seminars were organized and hired staff were sent to be trained. Ben admitted, "Unfortunately, there are less and less people willing to do voluntary work because many women now, married or single, are employed full time. So it's very difficult to get the number of persons volunteering but we do still have a hard core of persons who give of their time and service." Ben considered these early influences as fundamental to her later active involvement in the Student Nurses' Association where she and others arranged conferences, had 'shows' to raise money and were involved in the general well-being of the hospital, despite the daily twelve-hour tour of duty.

Ben has also held office at various levels in the Coterie, including the Port of Spain governing body. She was credited with proposing and facilitating the employment of a paid secretary. In 1984 she received the Distinguished Service Award from the organization. She has remained actively involved and, while not in office, has retained her membership. The year 1996 held much significance for the social history of the island and for Ben in particular. That year two women's institutions which changed the face of the nation celebrated their seventy-fifth anniversary. They also formed a central part of Ben's life. The Coterie of Social Workers and the founding of the Bishop Anstey High School meant that more black girls would be able to have a secondary education, albeit fee-paying. These two organizations made it possible for black women to be the movers and shakers for social progress for oppressed women and children in their island. In April 1996 yet another award was bestowed on Ben for her many contributions to the Coterie of Social Workers' San Fernando branch. Today, the Coterie's initial feeding of poor and malnourished schoolchildren in the 'breakfast sheds' has been incorporated by the government into a regular school feeding programme. Thousands of meals a day are served throughout the island with the Coterie and its many branches as the main supplier of these meals to the government.

Ben was also interested in politics. She was one of the founders of the League of Women Voters, a nonpartisan organization, but she has resisted joining a political party because she believes that she has been given opportunities for knowledge and experience that relatively few women had at that time. She did not want to be "harnessed by the fact that I have a loyalty to one party, that anybody in the community who came up to me and asked my opinion on something that I might have knowledge about, that I should be able freely and unfettered to give an honest opinion".

The League of Women Voters in Trinidad and Tobago was started in 1949 by Leonora Pujadus McShine. She had met a lawyer, Edith Bornn, from the US Virgin Islands who worked with the Caribbean Commission. Bornn introduced them to the idea of the League of Women Voters. They were informed about its existence in the United States, nonpartisan but political, and the advantages of forming such an organization. Leonora travelled from Port of Spain to San Fernando to meet with Ben to see if she would be interested in helping to form a similar league. This was in 1949, a time when full adult franchise had been granted and there would be elections. People were becoming increasingly politically awakened and women realized that, with their votes, they too would have their say in the political arena. Leonora and Ben were family friends so it was not surprising that she would consult with Ben. Leonora also knew that Ben was active in community projects and other groups. They shared similar interests and were "sort of criticizing things that were happening and thought it was time that we did something about it. Do we think, as a women's group, we could do something about it? That was the idea." Ben agreed with the concept, gathered a group of friends together and decided that they would enrol in a basic economics course. Ben pointed out, "The basis of all our political problems at that time was economic in the country." They formed the San Fernando Study Group in 1950 and later enrolled in an elementary economics course offered by the Extra-Mural Department of UWI. They not only attended classes but invited politicians and nonpolitical people to give guest lectures on a variety of topics. Meanwhile Leonora did the same in Port of Spain. The two separate groups eventually merged to form the National League of Women Voters, but they continued to have branches in the north and south of the island. Ben was chairman of the southern branch.

The objectives of the league were to interest women in the study of matters relating to government and to the social, economic and political conditions of the colony and adjacent areas; to educate women with regard to their responsibility to exercise the vote; to ensure the representation of women on committees and bodies, particularly those set up to advise on matters related to education, health, and the morals of the community; to examine legislation and its application to women, children and the home; and to render such services in the interest of education in citizenship as may be possible.[13]

Some of the important activities undertaken were educational, including preparation of booklets on the various arms of the government, such as *Knowing Your Government* and *Know Your County Council*, which explained the structure of the councils and the law, the nature of elections, candidates and other relevant subjects. The booklets, although designed for all, provided basic knowledge. Their prime purpose was to encourage women to become involved in politics. The league had pre-election forums held at the Town Hall where the public could question the candidates on their stands on issues. There were no parties as such, since it was still Crown government, so candidates ran as individuals representing a constituency. The forums were usually crowded, "with people standing outside". Ben told me that they undertook something that was unheard of at the time: "We used to hire microphones, put them on motorcars. You have no idea the sensation this caused in the 1940s . . . Those of us who had cars, we would go out with this microphone into all the districts . . . and stand on the street corners and tell the people . . . they must go out and vote, what they should do to vote, why it was their duty to vote. And they would come up and say 'When you finish speaking Miss we're going to vote for you.' And we said 'We're not up for election. We're not candidates. We don't want you to vote for us, we want you to know all the people who are going up for elections and make up your mind who can do what needs to be done in your area.' "

When party government came into being in 1956, the league did not support any particular party. One of the conditions of membership was that while individual members could belong to a party, they could no longer be an officer in the league. The league, among other movements, was very instrumental in preparing women for participation in party politics and it helped to propel women into politics. Some members of the league eventually became senators and members of the Legislative Council. Among them were Vern Critchlow, Ada Date Camps and Lynne Beckles who became leading members of the People's National Movement, a major nationalist party led by a brilliant intellectual, Dr Eric Williams.

Ben was adamant that she never wanted to become politically aligned, even when she was approached by one of the parties. This stance revealed her central core, her integrity, a term that was repeatedly used by colleagues to describe her. Although she was not involved in formal politics, Ben was for many years the national representative for the League of Women Voters.

One of Ben's major interests was her involvement with the Soroptimists. She is a chartered member of the Soroptimist International of Trinidad and Tobago. Audrey Jeffers, founder of the Coterie, was invited to establish this branch by the Soroptimist Organization in Britain. Members are recruited only by invitation, extended to professional or businesswomen who are in a position of leadership. The latter criterion has been somewhat modified in recent years and it now requires that the individual is knowledgeable and has the ability to speak for the particular group or category that is represented. The purpose of the organization is to improve the status of women internationally through goodwill and understanding. In Trinidad, in particular, it is concerned with the well-being of the country. There are committees dealing with a variety of aspects in the nation's business, such as politics, education, nutrition and citizenship. It is considered the female counterpart of Rotary. In 1950 Ben became a member of the Trinidad and Tobago Agricultural Society and magnanimously chose to represent agriculture as a businesswoman rather than a nurse, because "few women went into agriculture". She knew that if she represented nursing it would prevent anyone else in that discipline from becoming a member.

Ben is the administrator of the family estate, with a manager and staff, producing cocoa, coffee and bananas for export. She is considered to be a good financial manager who knows the money market. When she became chairman of the finance committee in the Soroptimists club, it was 'in the red'. Ben invested the money which generated income and brought the club back to a healthy financial condition. Louise Horne, retired nutrition officer for the Windward Islands, spoke highly of Ben's business acumen. "She could tell you about produce, prices, management of staff – a businesswoman, to the extent when we needed money she said, 'Let us get into the lottery business.' That was a long time ago and we are still in it. She was in charge of that."[14] She has represented the organization overseas at her own expense and was the president of Soroptimists International, Trinidad, from 1976 to 1977. On the occasion of their golden jubilee in 1984, the Soroptimists bestowed on her a service award.

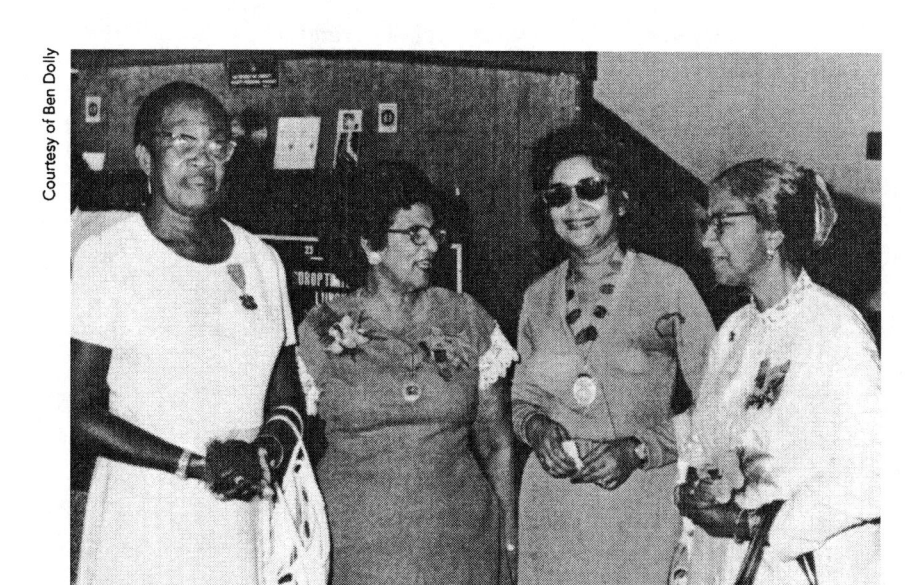

From left to right, Louise Horne, Merle Lutchman (master of ceremonies), Gemma Ramkissoon, Ben Dolly (president), Soroptimists International, 1976

In the early 1940s Ben had been one of the founders of the Chest and Heart Association in San Fernando. Originally, it had been called the Society for the Prevention of Tuberculosis and had been dormant for some time with the improvement in health standards. In 1952, however, Ben was approached by the governor's wife, Lady Rance, and asked to consider revisiting it. Ben gathered a group of interested parties and they started a centre. Their revised activities focused on rehabilitation and teaching crafts. Some financial aid was given to clients to assist in attending clinics, as well as counselling on lifestyle.

In addition to her voluntary work for a number of community and women's organizations, Ben has served in a number of government bodies. In the 1950s she was appointed to the prestigious Julien Commission concerned with health services in the nation. In the 1980s Ben served on a government committee that was established to prepare a report and conduct private and public consultations on tertiary education, training and research with representatives of UWI at St Augustine, with particular reference to the future direction of nursing education. The 1980s was a period when the university's role and functions were being challenged to be more relevant to the needs of the society and to embrace all the professions. Ben, together with the executive of the Trinidad and Tobago Registered Nurses' Association (TTRNA), including the current executive secretary, Yvonne Pilgrim, worked assiduously in preparing a brief for presentation to that committee.

She was also appointed to several non-health related committees. One was the Local Public Assistance Board in San Fernando, on which she served for a number of years. The board is responsible for 'poor relief' (a government supplement) and old age pensions. Later, she was appointed to the Central Assistance Board, the statutory governing body in Port of Spain. This kept her in touch with people from all walks of life in the community. When county councils were first established, members were appointed to the various councils, and Ben was appointed to the health committee of the Victoria County Council in the 1960s. It is worth noting that only in 1937 were enfranchised women given the right to sit on county councils and even then only a very small minority of propertied women qualified for selection. Fewer still were eligible to vote for the Legislative Council and women were not eligible for political office. Ben's service on the county council continued until changes came and members were elected. Other key government committees included the Attorney General's Committee on Law Reform and the Prisons Committee concerned with prison reform. She served on the latter committee from 1972 to 1980. During those years many honours came her way for her untiring devotion not only to nursing but also to the broader health and social concerns. In 1975, during International Women's Year, she received two awards, one from the San Fernando Borough Council and the other from the Business and Professional Women's Club. When Trinidad and Tobago became a republic in 1976, the government paid Ben the greatest tribute by awarding her the nation's highest honour, the Medal of Merit (Gold) of the Order of the Trinity.

Ben believes a leader is one who is able to influence others to help in the achievement of a goal. She said, "No person who is a leader successfully really does the thing always [by] herself or himself. It is done through other people. So it is that ability to influence people to have a similar goal and to work towards that goal, that I think defines good leadership." Leadership, for her, demanded education but more importantly dedication and risks, "because you are swimming against the tide". Indeed, she exemplified those qualities that she defined. Her deep sense of commitment and dedication to nursing continued to motivate her to be its gatekeeper from 1988 through to 1990. She represented the professional association as a member of the committee which was established by the government to plan and organize the transfer of nursing education from the apprenticeship system in the hospitals to the College of Nursing. During the transition, she played a major role in ensuring that nursing did not lose its identity by being absorbed by any of the existing structures within the National Institute for Higher Education, Research, Science and Technology (NIHERST). There were, for example, serious attempts to have nursing education established in the existing College of Health Sciences, which encompassed allied health programmes.

Yvonne Pilgrim confirmed what has been pointed out before and is an axiom of life in all societies – the value of social networks for achieving political ends. She observed that Ben "used her social contacts in order to ensure that the College of Nursing was set up as an entity and subsequently the (Nurses) Act was amended" to reflect that reality. Ben knew the chairman of the Board of Governors of NIHERST and, as Yvonne noted, "You know that a lot of decisions are taken outside of a boardroom in a social setting . . . she used her influence to ensure that the college was established. So having used the influence outside of the formal meeting, when we got into the formal meeting, we were able to get it through."[15]

Ben Dolly is a historian by nature if not by training. She has a remarkable memory for details. During our interviews, there were several calls from TTRNA regarding a number of constitutional matters and it was amazing to hear her cite the file numbers where the secretary could find the information from old files. This skill is so vital in this part of the world because often the oral recollection of events can lead to the retrieval of information. Ben was recognized for her mentoring in this area of historical documentation and record keeping. Several colleagues mentioned this characteristic. Dr Jean Grayson, former chief nursing officer, noted that "she had the habit of going back in history and that we should learn from that . . . This is one of the reasons that I too became interested in history."[16] Lynne Beckles, former registrar of the Nursing Council, commented, "She is one of the few women I know that appreciate old, historical documents . . . There was no report, no treatises, no theses on professional nursing that Ben didn't try to collect and store away. I think that I got my love of storing old documents from her."[17] Louise Hunte made a similar comment: "She is a person who keeps records. If someone asks, 'Could you tell me so and so?' she said, 'Alright, I will look and see.' She has her papers, her records . . . She's businesslike. She is not rushing to put herself forward. She is doing it firmly but quietly."

Ben expressed deep concern that modern nurses were not interested in the historical archives although present-day nurses are taught research. She is a repository of much of the nursing data, oral as well as written. It is hoped that she will pass this on to the association and to those who care about the history of nursing in the island.

The two-day marathon sessions of interviews ended with Ben lavishing praise on nurses. "I have come to appreciate nursing more and more as I've grown older. Several times my life has been saved by the service of nurses. I have had severe illnesses during my life and the absolute devoted care and attention that I received from nurses at all levels has made me eternally grateful and appreciate what it is really to be cared by nurses." Ben expressed some fear that those who were advocating a bachelor's degree programme in nursing as entry to practice may not have examined critically whether that was the best option for Trinidad. She expressed justifiable concerns about the future of professional nursing and the possibility of misunderstanding the intent of such a programme. As she has wisely put it, "The person entering the programme must be oriented to know . . . that they are being better prepared so that they can give better care, not that they can give no care. They are better prepared so that their level of care will be even higher . . . and will be better than their predecessors. Not that they will give no care and stand aside and let somebody else do it. That's the danger. That's my only fear." Is her fear justified? Only time will tell. The bachelor's degree as entry to practice is not yet a reality in Trinidad, but it is the trend in the Western world, and experience has shown that nursing education in Trinidad is highly influenced by the Western countries. Therefore, it would be vitally important when promoting changes to clearly and deliberately identify, preserve and integrate indigenous traditions and practices in nursing education and practice to meet the needs of the local society.[18] Nursing education in the past has always attempted to do so. One can only hope that her fears do not become a reality.

The *Trinidad Guardian* is the oldest and most respected newspaper in the island. In 1992 it celebrated its seventy-fifth anniversary. It is telling that this remarkable woman was selected as one of the distinguished "75ers" to be interviewed for the special issue published for the occasion. Ben Dolly was described as "this remarkable woman who saw nursing as a vocation, a calling, as well as an occupation" and who avowed that "people retire from jobs but not from a profession". She was also described as a woman of substance "who has lived up to her potential and a woman who at 75 years continues to develop that potential in herself and in hundreds of lives she has touched over the years".[19] A fitting tribute then and now.

What were the events and circumstances that gave rise to this rare woman? To turn to that will require a journey back in time.

Notes

1. B. Brereton, *A History of Modern Trinidad, 1783–1962* (London: Heinemann, 1981), 108–14, 115; G. Lewis, *The Growth of the Modern West Indies* (New York: Monthly Review Press, 1968), 201; see also J. Hezekiah, "The Development of Health Care Policies in Trinidad and Tobago: Autonomy or Domination?", *International Journal of Health Services* 19, no. 1 (1989): 82.
2. L. Brathwaite, "Social Stratification in Trinidad" *Social and Economic Studies* 2 (1953): 5–175.
3. E. Williams, *History of the People of Trinidad and Tobago* (Port of Spain, Trinidad: PNM Publishing, 1962), 216–25.
4. Lewis, *The Growth of the Modern West Indies*, 208.
5. O. Senior, *Working Miracles: Women's Lives in the English-speaking Caribbean* (Cave Hill, Barbados: Institute of Social and Economic Research, 1991), 104–28.
6. R.E. Reddock, *Women, Labour and Struggle in Twentieth Century Trinidad and Tobago, 1898–1960* (The Hague: Institute of Social Studies, 1984), 326–41, where she discusses women and women's organizations and struggles.
7. Lorna Rigsby, personal interview, February 1996. All material quoted from Rigsby is from this interview.
8. Joan Massiah, personal interview, April 1996. All material quoted from Massiah is from this interview.
9. Stephen Dolly, personal interview, April 1996. All material quoted from Stephen Dolly is from this interview.
10. Hilary Dolly, personal interview, April 1996. All material quoted from Hilary Dolly is from this interview.
11. K. Gibran, "On Marriage", *The Prophet* (New York: Knopf, 1961), 15–16.
12. Reddock, *Women, Labour and Struggle*; the Coterie was the organization that Dame Nita's uncle Dr O'Neal became involved with for many years during his stay in Trinidad. See chapters 1 and 7.
13. Reddock, *Women, Labour and Struggle*, 589.

14. Louise Horne, personal interview, March 1996. All material quoted from Horne is from this interview.
15. Yvonne Pilgrim, personal interview, March 1996. All material quoted from Pilgrim is from this interview.
16. Jean Grayson, personal interview, April 1996. All material quoted from Grayson in this chapter is from this interview.
17. Lynne Beckles, personal interview, April 1996. All material quoted from Lynne Beckles is from this interview.
18. J. Hezekiah, "The Development of Nursing Education in Trinidad and Tobago: 1956–1986" (PhD diss., University of Alberta, Edmonton, 1987), 258.
19. *Trinidad Guardian*, seventy-fifth anniversary edition, 30 August 1992, 37–38.

CHAPTER FOUR

Developing the Nursing Profession

Born in 1917 in the rural district of New Grant, in the southern part of Trinidad, Berenice was the eldest of three daughters of James Emmanuel Grant, a pharmacist. He was trained at the San Fernando Colonial Hospital where, in the 1800s, pharmacists paid a small fee for tuition and were taught the sciences by teachers from Scotland. Her mother, Mary Callistra, was a housewife who took an active role in village activities. She was a community-oriented person whom the villagers often sought out for advice regarding any ailment. The family also owned land and was involved in agriculture, but James Grant owned his own pharmacy. He was very active in the Pharmaceutical Society of Trinidad and Tobago, and became president of the group. Many of the pharmacists then went on to study medicine and, while he would have liked to do the same, it was beyond his means. At that time, pharmacists were licensed to practise under the Medical Board Ordinance, and he worked actively to have the Pharmacy Board Ordinance passed so that pharmacists could control their own licensure or registration. However, he died before it came into effect. Ben and her father spent much time discussing the issue of licensure since she had experienced the struggle for the Nurses Ordinance, similar to the pharmacists, as the practice of nursing also had formerly come under the control of the Medical Board Ordinance.

It was clear where Ben got her drive for independence, community and professional involvement. Both parents were role models. Moreover, she added,

"I was the first. So I think that this position of leadership and responsibility came from that, in that I was always made to feel that I was supposed to set the example ... There was no mistake about my responsibility in my family at all. I don't know if others accepted it." Her father was an Anglican and her mother Roman Catholic and the children were all brought up as Roman Catholics. Ben stressed, however, that although it was before the time of ecumenism, they lived, moved and worked among those of other faiths. The Anglican church was opposite where they lived and had been a part of her father's family estate until the Grant family had given the land to the church. Ben recalled going to Sunday school with friends of other faiths even though it was not permitted at that time.

The Grant children, Ben, Vera, her middle sister, and Lesley, the youngest, and their mother remained at home while James Grant travelled to work at his pharmacy, which was some distance away. The girls started early schooling where they lived near Princess Town. Then they were sent to board in Port of Spain for their elementary schooling at Tranquillity Girls' Intermediate School. Tranquillity was considered to be a prime elementary school because it combined a primary school curriculum with some secondary education. It was administered by the government, while others were under the auspices of the Roman Catholic church. The curriculum at Tranquillity was more extensive than at the basic elementary or primary schools and the teachers and headmistress were British. Ben boarded with friends of the family in Port of Spain initially, but she and her sisters spent most time with a widow, Mrs Pinheiro, and her daughter.

In 1928 Ben created history as she was the first girl in the island ever to come first in the College Exhibition Examination, which in colonial days automatically gave her a full scholarship to a high school. Trinidad's education system was very similar to that in Barbados, with few children going beyond primary school. The private secondary schools were fee-paying and scholarships were few. When Ben took the College Exhibition Examination, only eight government scholarships were available for the two islands. Given these conditions, it is remarkable that in 1928 Ben, a coloured girl from a middle-class family, not only completed primary schooling but became the top student, and the first girl, in the annual primary school examinations to win a scholarship which allowed her to obtain free secondary education.[1] Although Ben was accepted at St Joseph's Convent, the Roman Catholic girls' secondary school, she chose Bishop Anstey High School, an Anglican girls' secondary school. Many of her friends from Tranquillity Girls' School were going to Bishop Anstey and this influenced her choice. Moreover, St Joseph's Convent was still seen as the preserve of the white upper class with few blacks. There was much rejoicing over her achievement in the island by girls in general and in the Grant family in particular. The thrill of Ben's life was the gift of a bicycle by her proud parents.

Bishop Anstey High School, opened in 1921, was not only highly regarded but attracted more of the upper- and middle-class coloured and black girls. Ben lavished praise on the education she received there. The headmistress, a Miss Stevens, from Bristol in England, was "very strict, prim, you know the sort of Victorian type. But we are eternally grateful for the type of education we got. It taught us civic consciousness." The girls received a broad, all-round education. Ben recalled Miss Stevens asking them who had won the Nobel Prize, and getting them interested in the politics and elections of the island when the labour movement was evolving in the 1930s. Not only was the curriculum rich (Ben took science, mathematics and the arts) but the school's setting was unusually attractive. It was surrounded by high walls with a beautiful garden, ablaze with flowers, and the students were expected to know the names of all the trees and flowers in the garden. The most coveted prize of the school was not for academic performance but for general usefulness and leadership in school activities. It was called the Good Citizenship Prize and voted on by the teachers and senior students. Needless to say, Ben won that prize.

At about the age of fourteen, Ben became a member of the Girl Guides, and was soon a company leader. Through this movement, she met Dr and Mrs Metivier and went to their home, with other Guides, to prepare for the Girl Guide badges for nursing. Avis Metivier was a British registered nurse. She was very interested in the advancement of the nursing profession, as was her husband, a Trinidadian ophthalmologist. Between them they made great efforts to develop nursing education in the island. As in the other West Indian territories, the low status of nurses and their difficult working conditions meant that the profession attracted predominantly women of the lower middle class. Mrs Metivier, one of the founders of the Port of Spain Trained Nurses' Association, was very involved in her professional organization and because of this she was always looking for nursing recruits with a higher education than the average nurse of those days. She encouraged the young Girl Guides and taught them from her home. Proficiency badges were given in Guiding, such as sick nursing, child nursing, home nursing, first aid and domestic science. Ben became very involved in these activities which strongly influenced her final decision to enter nursing. She recounted, "In those days, of course, we were taught to help one another, but I think that the seed was sown in me long before that. I remember as a child, my sister and I were patients at the San Fernando Hospital. We were both there for a tonsillectomy. In those days, it was just a matter of staying in the hospital for a few days . . . We were so happy with the nurses, the day nurses and the night nurses, so that when our parents came for us we did not want to go home. I have always felt that something in the attitude of those nurses, their kindness, their caring, and the way we felt absolutely at home, in spite of the fact that we went there for a traumatic experience, had a profound influence on me. To me the hospital became a second home . . . Those happy memories removed the terror that children normally feel for hospitals . . . I've always remembered with gratitude those nurses. One of them is still alive, Nurse Ella Allen."

Bishop Anstey High School had a 'Big Sister' programme in which a younger student was mentored by a more senior student. Ben said that she "was put on to someone who became a real big sister to me and who is still my dearest friend, Ann Lumsden, who has now returned after having been in England for many years. She retired there . . . I think perhaps it's because she went into nursing that must have helped me to go into nursing too. She went in and did this abroad because she had relatives there." Many years later, in 1945, Ann Lumsden became the first Trinidadian, UK educated nurse, to be appointed sister tutor to the colonial hospital in San Fernando. She turned a new leaf in nursing education as it was the first time in Trinidad that a sister tutor was not on contract to the Colonial Office. In Ann, Ben indeed had an excellent mentor and role model.

Ben graduated from Bishop Anstey by completing the Cambridge Examinations which were administered from England. She matriculated in the Senior Cambridge, a feat of no small significance for a girl in the 1930s. Mrs Metivier was very impressed by Ben. She actively pursued the possibility of Ben becoming a nurse by approaching the matrons of the two major colonial hospitals, the Port of Spain Hospital and the San Fernando Hospital, and arranging interviews for Ben with each of the matrons. Ben was accepted by both hospitals. She chose the San Fernando Hospital since it was nearer to home. Even though Ben received her secondary education in Port of Spain in the north, she strongly identified with the south. As she remarked, "My real home was always in the south . . . We are southerners, but Port of Spain is just as familiar to me."

Ben's father was not pleased with his daughter's choice of career, but her mother supported her decision. Ben noted that her father felt, "There were other things that I could do, but the hospital called. I think he had the idea that nursing was a subordinate profession. He didn't say so in so many words, but looking back, I think he felt that the sky was the limit, that I could achieve as I had the ability to achieve and he didn't place a value on nursing. Hardly anybody did in those days. He felt that it wasn't good enough and that I should do something better." It was not clear what occupation he had hoped his daughter would choose. As was the case elsewhere, for the majority of middle- and upper-middle-class women the only possibilities for employment were in teaching, nursing and midwifery or as druggists and junior staffers in the civil service. Perhaps he had hoped Ben would enter teaching, for that was by far the most important means for social mobility for black and coloured women and was held in greater esteem than nursing.[2] He also thought that because Ben's education was superior to that of the vast majority in nursing she would not be able to submit to the authority of the senior nurses or subordinate herself to the rigours of the discipline. Ben quoted him as saying, "When you go, it is your mistake, I want you to remember that I had no part in it."

Ben has never regretted entering the profession and remained eternally grateful to "all the older nurses who I know did not perhaps have the same advantages I had in their basic education. But they were wonderful people. People of great character, people of great caring, and they had much to teach me. So I enjoyed working with them and learning from them."

Becoming a Nurse

During the 1920s and 1930s a succession of English matrons were in charge of the hospitals. This contributed to a gradual deterioration in nurses' training. Probationers worked for six months without pay so that their suitability for nursing could be determined. The conditions of work and the remuneration were comparable to those in Barbados and the other West Indian territories, except for an additional year for midwifery. By the early 1930s the increasing demands on the hospitals caused medical and nursing services to become strained, while at the same time the educational levels of applicants were unsatisfactory. Consequently, in 1935, a special board consisting of representatives of the directors of education and health was appointed to examine all applicants for admission. The obvious need for revision of the whole training of nurses began to receive attention.[3]

Ben began her training in 1937, with a batch of nine probationers. Nursing students were admitted haphazardly during the course of the year and their numbers varied dependent on the needs of the hospital at any given time. Recalling the long-sleeved uniform, with its large headpiece and stiffly starched, pleated apron and skirt, she said, "The uniform gave you a sense of propriety... and made you feel careful. You respected people and they respected you. Discipline becomes a part of you." Her parents and her schooling had already inculcated a sense of discipline and the rigour and formality of the programme reinforced this early training.

When Ben entered nursing, the training was three years for general nursing and an additional year for midwifery. It was not until 1938 that the first sister tutor from the Overseas Nursing Service was appointed to the Port of Spain Hospital. A revised syllabus and programme of training was started in 1943, two years after Ben had completed her training. She recalled that "in those days we did not really think of becoming a nurse or midwife to secure positions in the hospital because they did not exist for local nurses..You really trained to become an independent professional woman, because midwives in Trinidad held a very respected position in the community. I think that's more a French heritage, midwives. And of course, it was a little mystique that they could do things that doctors could do too, you know." Independent practice as a nurse and midwife afforded greater prestige as well as freedom from the rigidity and class system prevailing in the hospitals. Moreover, the midwifery programme was well established and renowned. It was due to its reputation that Nita Barrow went to Trinidad to gain experience in midwifery. Because there was no registration for nurses, they were not considered to be 'a nurse' until they became a midwife. The fact that nurses and midwives were trained side by side for many years is attributed to the belief that a nurse must also become a midwife. It could also be argued that the difference in public image and status was because midwifery had a long and well-respected past, while nursing registration occurred much later. It was not until the 1960s that a registered nurse no longer needed to be a midwife in order to practise.

It is worth noting that the hospitals at that time were staffed primarily by English nurses as matrons and sisters. The local staff were at the bottom of the

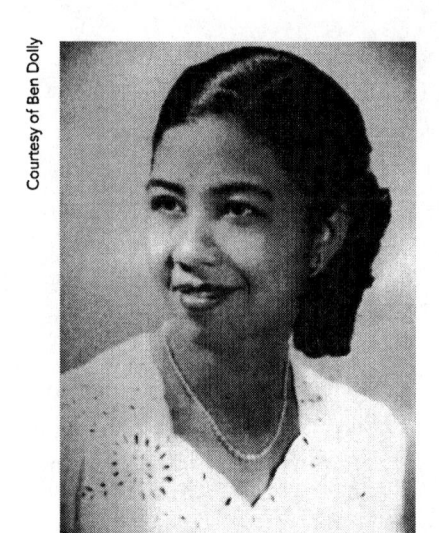

Ben Dolly, prior to entry into nursing, 1936

Courtesy of Ben Dolly

hierarchy either as students or staff nurses. Local nurses who worked in the hospitals often remained there for years without promotion and although they functioned in responsible positions, they were not appointed to senior positions. Many of these older women of great ability and character would be in charge when the British sisters went on leave. The unfairness of such practices did not go unheeded.

One of the contradictions of colonialism, and similar government systems, is that there are always individuals in the dominant group who rise as champions for the oppressed members. Through the efforts of Dr and Mrs Metivier and the English matron of the San Fernando Hospital, Miss Isabella Ristori, local nurses were eventually promoted from basic staff nurses to ward sisters. Mrs Metivier and Miss Ristori made representations to the government through the Nurses' Association to agitate for the advancement of local nurses. Eventually, in the late 1930s, local nurses were promoted to ward sisters.

Ben and her batch of student nurses were taught by the matrons and the medical officers. Ben stated, very pragmatically, "They were not persons trained in nursing education, but this is not peculiar to the Caribbean . . . The fact was that was the situation worldwide." At the San Fernando Hospital, there was only a small hostel which accommodated six people, so most probationers had to find their own accommodation. Ben lived with relatives in San Fernando and walked to the hospital early in the morning as she had to be on duty at six o'clock. She walked back home at night. She observed, "There wasn't even a bus service. It was during our studentship that a bus service came into San Fernando for the first time . . . The hospital held such a position in people's minds that when bus service came, they gave the student nurses strips of tickets to travel free on the bus."

Although the programme was arduous, the students enjoyed it. Ben had the distinction of winning the Princess Mary Silver Medal for Proficiency in Nursing Practice and Excellence in the nursing examinations. She was the youngest nurse to do so and she travelled to Port of Spain to receive her award. Ben reminisced: "My main memories of it are that those days were happy. We enjoyed one another's company. We enjoyed the hardships. We didn't think in terms of how much you were doing and how little you were getting. It didn't arise. I remember a particular incident once because our hospital was up on a hill and we could look down and see people going to work at eight o'clock in the morning to the business places. And I remember clearly going through my mind the thought that they did not realize how much time they had already wasted. We had worked for two hours and they were just going! They seemed to have wasted so much time . . . I think it was because the people with whom we worked were senior people who were so dedicated to their work."

Ben expressed some disillusionment about nursing today and attributed it primarily to the fact that students are allowed to be married while they are pursuing their studies. Although she was an ardent advocate for the rights of women, she contended that married nursing students experience much conflict and difficulty in trying to cope with the responsibilities inherent in both raising a family and learning the discipline. Regretfully, she said, "I'm sorry I have to admit this, but I do feel so, because there are certain vocations, I would call it, in which one has to be totally absorbed to perform properly. To have another vocation, in which you should be totally absorbed . . . I think that a lot of deterioration has taken place. I think that it is too hard for a student of nursing to really carry out responsibilities of a home and little babies getting ill and all that, and have this all absorbing profession . . . As a young student it is too stressful . . . In your student training you have to do certain things at a certain time. If you don't then your career stays back . . . Eventually it meant that many got lost to the profession – when she breaks her contract through circumstances in which she has no control, she sets back her whole life sometimes . . . and never makes it up at all and never enters the profession. It has happened to several people."

She buttressed her viewpoint with comments from married nursing students who stated, "We can't take it. There's too much pressure in the work and pressure in the home." At the time that Ben entered and completed training, married women were not allowed to enter nursing or even to continue in their jobs. It was therefore not surprising that Ben would echo the prevailing norm, although she was supportive of married women working. She allowed, "Once a person is qualified and she is a professional woman, she can organize her life and her time." And indeed she lived up to this philosophy. "I said straight that I wanted to be a nurse and that I intended to be a nurse, and that I was not getting married until I had finished my training. And this is what I did."

Ben left government service at the end of her training, and went on to take a health visitor's course, which is similar to a public health nursing course. It was a one-year programme, administered through the Royal Sanitary Institute in England. The examinations were held in a different West Indian island each year. This was before the West Indies School of Public Health was established in Jamaica with Nita Barrow as the head. Forever visionary and forward thinking, Ben said, "Nursing takes place where the client is. It does not have to be in the hospital . . . I say to nurses that they must stop being prisoners in the hospital . . . Taking health care and health facilities into the community, and meeting with other people and letting them know what nurses know and who they are. It's because nurses tend to . . . be prisoners in the institution, that the public as a whole does not recognize their value. They must get involved in things outside and take their knowledge and skills . . . because nursing by its very nature is progressive. It exposes you to all forms of life activity. But except you meet people outside, they don't notice, or don't respect your knowledge and ability." Indeed, today this concept that she espoused is receiving greater attention in North America as health care reform has caused hospitals to reduce their nursing staff. Community care is becoming the focus instead of hospital care. The frustration of local nurses in not having their knowledge and skills acknowledged or recognized by promotion, and in being treated like second-class citizens in the hospitals in their own country may well have been a factor in Ben's decision to work in the community, "where I used my knowledge and skills". She added, "Even a person like Dame Nita couldn't get into a senior position in the hospital. That is why she left Barbados after her basic training. She came here to do midwifery and then on to Canada and so on, because she could not get out of this rut as long as there was the colonial system."

Notwithstanding this, Ben and other nurses who were not employed in the hospitals were called upon to do voluntary work in the hospitals during the war years. They readily responded. All of Ben's contributions to nursing have been on a voluntary basis. She claimed that "the fact that it was not for remuneration is perhaps why some people say I'm not a nurse. It's funny, some nurses say that I'm not nursing . . . but the whole community knows me as a nurse." This is an interesting observation about nurses and nursing. Many nurses today, worldwide, still hold a view of nursing that is illness oriented and hospital based. Indeed, many people in the general population share a similar view. Yet as far back as Florence Nightingale, the role of the nurse in health promotion and illness prevention in the community has always been important in society but not readily acknowledged to be as vital as work in the hospital. It was especially noteworthy that the nature of Ben's work in the community, coupled with the fact that she was not paid for doing so, led to her contributions being devalued as not really being nursing by some. This phenomenon was akin to the role of the housewife or homemaker whose contributions to the well-being of the home and family were devalued and considered to be non-work because she was not paid for her efforts.

Very early in her training, Ben became involved in the student nurses' organization. She praised Isabella Ristori, the matron of the San Fernando Hospital. She was in charge when Ben was in training and, despite being a 'colonial', was very interested in the development of the profession in the island and of the quality of nursing care. Miss Ristori was instrumental in guiding and encouraging the young student nurses who, she felt, would carry on the professional ideas and ideals. She initiated and fostered the growth of the student nurses' organization in which she demonstrated further her leadership ability. It was a logical and natural progression that on graduation, Ben would become involved with her professional organization.

Visionary and Unifier

In June 1930 the trained nurses in the south of the island banded together in San Fernando to form the South Certificated Nurses' Association. The inaugural meeting was held on 2 July 1930. Mrs Marion Walls, a Canadian public health nurse and the wife of a Presbyterian missionary, Dr V.B. Walls, was elected president. In January 1932 the association's name was changed to the Certificated Nurses' Association of Trinidad and Tobago. The Port of Spain Trained Nurses' Association was inaugurated in March 1932 and in May expanded to include midwives, becoming the Port of Spain Trained Nurses and Midwives' Association. Their first president was Mrs Jessie Masson, followed later by Mrs Avis Metivier and then Mrs Ivy Waterman. There were now two organizations representing nurses, and it should be noted that only British or Canadian nurses were in the leadership positions in both associations. It would take Ben years to achieve the goal of unity.

Both the northern and southern associations were active in making representations to the local authorities as well as to the several committees and royal commissions that conducted enquiries into matters affecting nursing. As Ben observed, "It seems so silly for us to be holding out with two little groups of nurses appearing before the Moyne Commission for the Colonial Office, representing the same sort of people, and it came to my generation to do something about it." There had always been some sensitivity on the part of people in the south of the island, San Fernando, vis-à-vis those in the northern capital, Port of Spain. There were strong feelings on the part of the southern nurses that by joining with the north "everything will go to Port of Spain", and that San Fernando would be "left behind" in the proposed amalgamation. The southern nurses felt that they were the pioneers in forming an association. While both groups worked vigorously at promoting state registration for nurses, this separation did not bode well for hastening the process. Much guidance and assistance was given by members of the medical profession who were supportive of the idea of the nursing profession moving forward because, as Ben commented, "The medical profession was in the same situation where they also had to put up with inept people coming from the Colonial Office and being in top positions . . . [although] they didn't have to have a higher standard of training or education to get those positions." Dr James Waterman, Ivy's husband, was particularly helpful in the preparatory work for nurse registration.

Ben was an active member of the southern association from 1941, when "the very day that I joined I was made the secretary and I've never been out of office since." Ben continued, "I have never asked anybody to lead them, so anything that I have done, has been conferred only by my colleagues, people who were superior to me, both in the knowledge of nursing and the practice of it, my seniors in every way. They put me in positions of leadership and they kept me there . . . they have worked all along. People have worked with me [on] things that I have been credited with. We are the achievements of a lot of people behind the scenes. You know it is true there is a hard core like there is in every organization everywhere. I have been fortunate in that people, as I say, have given me positions of leadership . . . Kept me there for one reason or another, even though I knew they were dead against some of the things I believed in."

The importance of being a unified body was farsighted, as Ben pointed out, "You could not go and ask the government for an act for one area of the country. It was very important to be one body. One unified body." A visionary, she advocated combining the two associations, as "it was more important to have a professional association for the whole country than just a district of it".

It was not, however, until 1946, after exhaustive negotiations, that the two groups combined forces to become the Trained Nurses and Midwives' Association of Trinidad and Tobago (TNMATT), with a northern and a southern branch. It was not a happy occasion for those in the south who did not support the notion of combination. In fact, Marion Walls resigned. However, the union was a significant event as it heralded an era of combined efforts on plans and programmes that formerly had been fragmented.[4] The principal officers of the Joint Nursing Council for the unified association were Ben, as its first president, Ivy Waterman (British) as vice president, and Irene Mitchell, a Trinidadian nurse and one of the founders of the northern branch, as secretary treasurer. The Joint Nursing Council consisted of nine members, five from one branch and four from the other, determined on the basis of membership. Ben claimed that it had remained a loose arrangement (rather like a federation) in order to succeed. For example, the Port of Spain association decided to work towards a rest home for nurses and set up a fund for that purpose. Each branch had to function separately yet unite for international purposes, such as joining the ICN. Another major accomplishment of the joint association was the continuing publication of a biannual journal, initiated in 1945 by the Port of Spain branch.

Throughout the 1940s nurses vigorously pursued the quest for state registration. It was not an easy task. All midwives were already registered and licensed by the Medical Board, so that any proposed nursing act would need to have the knowledge and consent of the Medical Board since all practising nurses were also midwives. Considerable negotiating skills were required to work with members of both the Medical Board and the nursing association. Medical practitioners were always members of the fledgling association both when the nursing association was operating as two separate entities and when they combined. Drs Waterman, Francis and Innes were standing members. Ben recalled that when a delegation from the nurses' association met with the Medical Board in May 1944 to discuss the possibility of registration, the physicians could not comprehend why nurses needed registration. The usual patriarchy persisted, as they asked, "Why don't you want to be in the medical profession?" The contradictions in the attitude of local physicians were evident. While they wanted control of their own profession and positions of leadership in the health services within the colonial situation, they were reluctant to allow nurses similar autonomy. Like their colonial masters and predecessors, they wanted to be in control of nurses, yet paradoxically they sincerely wanted local nurses to occupy leadership positions in the health services, as long as medicine's undisputed authority over nurses was not threatened. Ben continued, "So we said, 'If you will not give us the midwife, well then we will have the registration without the midwives and you can keep the midwives.' That is how we eventually resolved it to get the [nursing] registration."

Ben, through her 'unstructured' research, had discovered that in England the majority of nurses were registered nurses but were not midwives as well. Consequently, the nurses' delegation recommended that nurses would stay with the medical profession as midwives but they wanted their own Nurses' Registration Act. Ben quoted Dr Innes as saying, "Stop it! You don't understand how we feel about nurses. We just don't want to let you go!" Their paternalism was apparent and not readily overcome. As well as working with the medical profession for registration, the nurses also had to obtain permission from the Colonial Office in

London. The nurses' gender and status as primarily women in relation to physicians who were primarily men, their having the lower status of the two disciplines, and the fact that they were black women seeking autonomy from the colonial structure presented a prime example of race, class and gender intersections. Applying directly to the Colonial Office in England could certainly facilitate matters. By chance, in 1947 Ben was travelling on holiday to England with her husband and family. She seized the opportunity to visit the Colonial Office and meet key officials there to present the association's case for independent nurse registration.

The pursuit of state registration for nurses was consistent with the report of the Rushcliffe Committee, which advocated local training with standards that would enable reciprocity with state registration in Great Britain. The Rushcliffe Committee had been appointed to examine both the training of British nurses for service in the colonies and the training of local nurses in the colonies. The need for post-registration training overseas, the introduction of the 'block' system of training,[5] and the appointment of at least one qualified and experienced sister tutor in training schools were among some of the major recommendations of the report. Three factors constrained the government in providing a series of scholarships. One was that further constitutional changes were occurring during the 1930s and 1940s; the second was the numerous recommendations from various reports; and finally, there were repeated requests for scholarships from the professional association. Consequently, by 1945 four student nurses were awarded scholarships to pursue basic training in the United Kingdom. Subsequently, scholarships for postgraduate training were awarded to six ward sisters who were selected for one-year courses in nursing education or nursing administration, or both, at the Royal College of Nursing and selected hospitals in the United Kingdom.[6]

Meanwhile, the British nursing sisters in Trinidad felt threatened by local nurses wanting to become registered nurses like themselves. A group of them wrote a letter to the secretary of state for the colonies stating that the nurses who wanted to call themselves registered nurses were not worthy to be recognized as such because they had training only up to the preliminary level.

Undeterred by this action, the association continued working on several fronts. It was instrumental in providing scholarships in 1944 and 1945 for local nurses to continue their education in public health at the West Indies School of Public Health in Jamaica. This move subsequently resulted in the government offering scholarships for postgraduate studies. The association had to "beg, borrow, subscribe and have functions" to raise the money for the constrained government to provide a series of scholarships. There were tea parties, donations and 'flag' days when they sold nurses' association flags. Ben reflected, "In those days it seemed like a mountain of money, you know. I think it cost us nearly a thousand dollars. A thousand dollars then was like a million now. Because nurses were working for thirty and forty dollars a month. And we raised the money." A strong sense of commitment and determination informed the actions of the nurses of that era in pursuit of their professional enhancement. They were dedicated to the goal of transferring nursing leadership into their own hands. This was the postwar era which saw the introduction of full adult franchise in the country in 1946 and the first elections held under universal suffrage, the maturation of the trade union movement, and the intensification for self-government and Federation. The universal mood was for taking control of all island affairs and for West Indian unity. Nurses, too, shared that mood and belief in the future.

Briefs were prepared for presentations, led by Ben, to the many Colonial Office committees, particularly the MacManus Nursing Commission. In 1947 Emily MacManus, matron of Guy's Hospital, London, and Blanche Shenton, an English public health nurse, visited Trinidad as part of assignment from the Colonial Office in order to report on the organization, training, and registration of those engaged in nursing the sick in the British West Indian territories. Their report dealt at length with poor conditions, facilities for training, and the need for better training. Unlike the reports produced by other commissions of inquiry, there was no written support for the assumption of ultimate responsibility by local nurses. Notwithstanding this, MacManus gave much encouragement, inspiration and assistance to the nurses at the numerous meetings held during her visit to the island, and was of invaluable help in discussing the proposed law for registration of nurses.[7]

The TNMATT continued its intensified pressure for the granting of state registration. On every occasion that Ben travelled to Britain with her husband and family on overseas leave, she represented her professional association to a number of different nursing organizations. She did what she termed 'unstructured research' to find out more about the process of professional registration. In 1947 she visited the General Nursing Council and spent a few days there observing the organization, and its filing system, and studying the Nurses' Act, noting how discipline of nurses was carried out. She also attended disciplinary meetings and council meetings. She then visited the Central Midwives' Board, the Colonial Office and the Overseas Nursing Association to collect as much information as she possibly could. She also visited the Royal College of Nursing to discuss setting up post-basic courses to meet the needs of the local nurses. Mrs Ivy Waterman used part of her leave to go to Edinburgh, where she had formerly been a matron, to try to secure places that would accept Trinidadian nurses for further education. The first nurses to benefit from those initiatives left Trinidad for Scotland in 1948.

This thrust, spearheaded by Ben, for furthering the nurses' professional practice and education as well as the standards of the profession was recorded in the journal of the association in its October 1947 issue:

Both the President and the Vice President (Mrs Dolly and Mrs Waterman) of our Association have returned from a long holiday in Great Britain ... Miss Udell Grant (Chief Nursing Officer at the Colonial Office, London) was interviewed and many interesting points were raised and discussed and visits were made to the Colleges of Nursing in London and Edinburgh, the Queen's District Nursing Association in London, Public Health Departments, Day Nurseries and Child Welfare Clinics. At all, an assurance was given that any of our nurses would be given help and encouragement if they proceeded for postgraduate studies in the UK. The need for our registration was stressed.[8]

By 1948 the government appointed a committee to examine the question of state registration for nurses. The committee was under the chairmanship of Dr A. Peat, director of medical services, Dr A. Francis, Dr H. Gillette, and five nurses, Olive Dwyer, Irene Montenegro, Lillian Seymour, Ivy Waterman and Ben. From 1948 to 1950 Ben and Ivy's roles as president and vice president were reversed until Ben again assumed the presidency mantle in 1950. The contribution of the association, under the stewardship of Ben Dolly and Ivy Waterman, to nursing education cannot be underestimated. They worked hard at improving the status of nursing. Dr James Waterman and Dr Aldwyn Francis, Office of the Director of Medical Services, are credited with providing assistance, guidance and leadership to the association during the 1940s when it was struggling, and their support continued for many years. Their interest in the education of nurses and in the excellence of nursing care for patients inspired the organization to maintain the struggle when all efforts seemed to end in frustration. Dr Waterman assisted the leadership in preparing the first draft of the nurses' ordinance for state registration.

When the bill was being debated at Government House, nurses took time off from duty from the then colonial hospital in Port of Spain. Words of encouragement were proffered to them, during an adjournment of the debate, by the Honourable Roy Joseph, member for the borough of San Fernando, who had presented the bill to the House in a lengthy and impassioned speech. He had been an ardent advocate in the House for many years in defence of the rights of nurses. In his speech to the House he noted that, with registration, it would then be possible for nurses to be eligible for full acting allowances and even for appointment to the post of nursing sister. He commented cynically, "I would not say, Your Excellency, that the reason for delaying action on the matter was to deny local nurses the right to get full acting allowances or to become Nursing Sisters."[9]

It was because of the vision, dedication, fortitude and perseverance of those nurses, led by Ben, that the Nurses' Registration Ordinance No. 38 was finally passed in June 1950. It received royal assent in December 1950. Subsequently the Nursing Council of Trinidad and Tobago was established, the first nursing council in the West Indies. (Barbados already had a Nurses' Registration Act from as early as 1932, but, as Ben stated, "There was no question of the nursing profession running their own affairs.") The Nursing Council of Trinidad and Tobago was the culmination of almost two decades of struggle and frustration for local nurses and midwives to gain professional status in their own right.

Pearl Peters, a colleague whom Ben 'roped in' to join the association in the early 1940s, asserted that it was Ben's fight for the nurses of Trinidad and Tobago to be professionally recognized and have a nursing council that was her lasting contribution. In Pearl's words, "Because there were so many people calling themselves nurses and they were not qualified so she kept drumming into the nurses' heads that you must fight for registration . . . she was in the forefront."[10]

Realizing a Dream

The Bill for Registration of Nurses was passed and the Nursing Council of Trinidad and Tobago together represented a milestone in the history of nursing and nursing education in Trinidad and Tobago, and indeed in the region. For this major accomplishment, much credit must be given to the leadership of Ben and the nurses' association which continued undaunted in pursuit of obtaining nurse registration. Lynne Beckles, secretary of the Nursing Council, now retired, said of Ben, "Mrs Dolly was an institution in her own right. It was her drive and persistence that persuaded the powers that be to create the Nursing Council of Trinidad and Tobago under which nurses could be registered. But the active participation in the movement to create a council, I would say it was almost, 99⅔ percent of Ben Dolly. She had . . . a singleness of purpose that I admired and you don't find it now in the young people. Roy Joseph was the member of parliament for her area and she got his ear . . . She would never take the president leader's role. She'd leave the presidency to somebody else but she would be the driving force behind it."[11]

The issue of social class inevitably rears its head in discussion of most, if not all, issues in the country. Ben was of the same social class as Roy Joseph and she would meet him at events, at meetings, visits or other occasions, and he became very interested in the nurses' cause. Lynne explained, "Now, if there were this big social gap, she could not have done that. Right? And she got him interested and he piloted the bill and got it passed." This observation was corroborated by others who pointed out that middle and upper income elite women, because of their connections, had access to decision-making centres of the political process and were good channels for gaining support. (Nita Barrow was another example of this useful social interaction.)

An interim council was formed, consisting of eight representatives of the TNMATT. It comprised Ben, two persons nominated by the governor in council, two nominated by the Medical Board, and three members of the association, who were appointed to conduct the affairs of the council for two years. In that time they were to set up the first register, prepare for the first election of a council under the ordinance, and draw up the rules and regulations for the council. Their first task was to differentiate between those nurses who had completed a recognized basic nursing programme and received a government certificate, and those who had not fully completed a programme or written a final examination but had worked in a hospital or the community for some time. Those with a certificate were put on the first register. The others had to provide evidence of having worked either in a district hospital or with a private practitioner under some form of supervision. They were put on a list called existing practitioners. Gradually, after a number of years, the council was able to close that list as the intent was only to 'grandfather' those existing practitioners who were practising at the time that registration came into being. These activities were all financed by the association until the council was able to organize its own affairs. The council eventually assumed responsibility for the syllabus and the examinations for nursing education – functions that were performed by the hospitals for many decades.

The first president of the Nursing Council was Ivy Waterman; Ben was vice president. Lynne Beckles said of Ben, "She would stay in the background and lead and direct . . . a great democrat, that woman . . . She would never do anything unless it was put to the council or the opinion of the members. She was very, very good at that sort of thing . . . What we admired about her was her unblemished integrity. Ben was honest to a fault . . . she could not be devious or lie, not Ben Dolly. She would rather tell you the nasty truth rather than lie."

Ben was a member on several committees of the council where she initiated the development of a number of administrative policies that are still effective and operational at the present time. Lynne was grateful that Ben was insistent that the various committees kept to their terms of reference and dealt exclusively with only those issues that were relevant to their domain. Her advice facilitated a smooth and more efficient functioning of council's activities. The first nursing examinations by the council were held in November 1951, and yet another new page in the history of nursing education was turned, with Ben playing a pivotal role in this transition.

In 1951 Jamaica was also seeking to get their nurse registration so that there was close communication between the two countries, and also with Guyana. The expertise of Julie Symes, a British nursing sister, who became Jamaica's first registrar, was most helpful to the nurses of Trinidad. Of those years of hard work towards registration, Ben commented, "We were in touch with Nita Barrow when she left Trinidad as a member of the Port of Spain Nurses' Association . . . Nita was one of the moving spirits in Jamaica . . . the difference, perhaps, in the struggle in the two territories at that time was that it was a struggle fought in Trinidad by Trinidad and Tobago nurses, trained and educated here; the persons who were leaders in Jamaica, many of them trained abroad. So it was much easier for them to get recognition with the public." This point of view could be subject to dispute; notwithstanding, it was a struggle for both associations to obtain their registration. In 1956, at a conference of the TNMATT, a resolution was passed changing the name of the association to the TTRNA, with northern and southern branches.

By 1955 the government had recognized that the Nursing Council was functioning effectively. Consequently, the director of medical services asked the council to consider assuming responsibility for the registration of midwives. While midwives had been examined and given

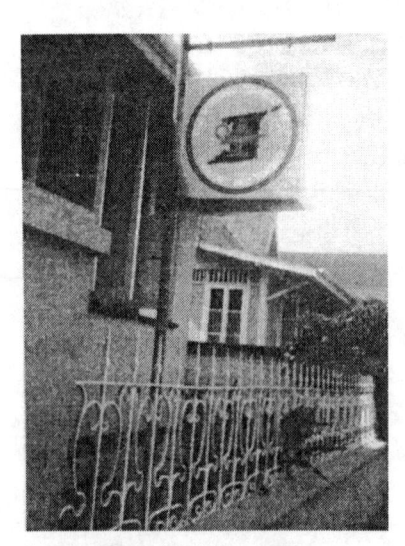

Nursing Council Building, 1979

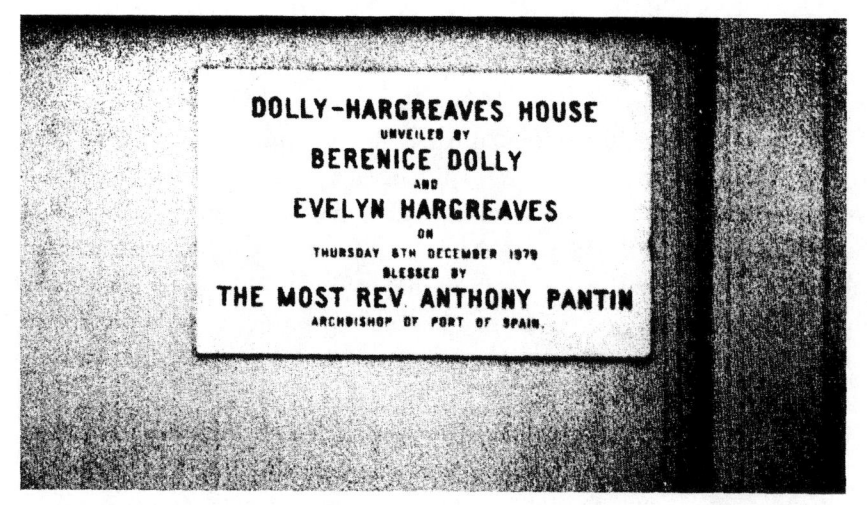

> **DOLLY-HARGREAVES HOUSE**
> UNVEILED BY
> **BERENICE DOLLY**
> AND
> **EVELYN HARGREAVES**
> ON
> THURSDAY 6TH DECEMBER 1979
> BLESSED BY
> **THE MOST REV. ANTHONY PANTIN**
> ARCHBISHOP OF PORT OF SPAIN.

Plaque, Dolly-Hargreaves Building, 1979

certificates by the Medical Board since 1935, there was no maintenance or regulation of their activities. Acquiring this function was quite a coup for the council, as the Nurses' Ordinance was amended to include midwives on the register in 1960, and the Nursing Council assumed responsibility for the training and examination of midwives.

When the council moved into its own quarters on 6 December 1979, as testament to Ben's dynamic leadership in the achievement of registration for nurses, the building was named after her and the president of the council at that time – the Dolly-Hargreaves Building.

THE QUEST – THE INTERNATIONAL COUNCIL OF NURSES

In 1949 the TNMATT had applied for membership of the ICN, the worldwide umbrella organization for all professional nursing organizations that meet certain prescribed standards. The successful realization of registration of nurses in Trinidad and Tobago did not go unnoticed. On the basis of this achievement, the ICN appointed Ben, then president of the association, the national representative for Trinidad and Tobago at their board of directors meeting in Brussels in 1951. In addition, the association was invited to the international congress in Rio de Janeiro in June 1953. It was here that the association was admitted to full membership of the ICN. Ben credited the idea of joining the ICN to Miss Ristori, the former matron of the San Fernando Hospital, who had long since left the island. Miss Ristori was a Florence Nightingale scholar and, as Ben remembered, "she had this book, which I have somewhere . . . it is a historical document . . . she had left this book with us, *The ICN*, . . . so this was her idea of [our] becoming international nurses. We had no idea what it was about." So they soon recognized the added value of being registered. To become a member of the ICN is prestigious for a nursing organization, since membership informs the nursing world that nurses from that country are registered and have an internal body to monitor standards of practice and education.

Ben continued to use her political, interpersonal and advocacy skills to facilitate and ensure that association would gain full admittance to the ICN. They invited ICN delegates passing through Trinidad on their way to the congress to stay at the homes of Trinidadian nurses. The local nurses met their in-transit colleagues at the airport and some members accepted their hospitality either on the way to Brazil or on their return flight. Ben shared some of the complexity involved with this final stage of achieving recognition by the ICN. On the plane to Brazil, Ben was invited to sit with the president of the Canadian delegation who pointed out to her the chairman of the ICN membership committee and suggested that Ben talk with her, an opportunity Ben immediately seized. That chairman was Florence Emory, an eminent Canadian nurse and the president of the Registered Nurses' Association of Ontario. Ben claimed that it was a privilege to have met and conversed with her because of her experience and knowledge of international affairs. Ben recollected, "She said, 'Your application is here?' And I said 'Yes.' And she said, 'Well you have a good chance but there are two problems we don't understand. One is that you have this joint executive committee. You have to have one nursing association.' I said, 'Yes, but we formed ourselves into one association, into this group, because it was not easy for two existing organizations to completely integrate right away. So we formed this and we do everything on a national basis in that committee.'"

The second problem was the fact that membership in the association included midwives who were not registered nurses. On her arrival in Brazil, Ben contacted Pearl Peters in Trinidad, an officer of the association, by telephone and cable. Ben knew she could trust Pearl to do everything in her power to forward to her immediately the information regarding the number of midwives on the register. Pearl went through the registration membership and "sent down the numbers for me... I presented them and they were satisfied that it was a group that was petering out... We could not exclude them from the association when this new concept arrived. They were the persons who formed the association in the days when midwifery was the only legally recognized qualification in this country... I said, 'They are a very small group and as they die off, we are not going to take anybody like that again.'... They accepted that and we were handed the membership on the 2nd July 1953 in Brazil." Ben's official reply at the admission of the TNMATT into full membership of the ICN was as follows:

Madam President,

May I on behalf of the Registered Nurses of Trinidad and Tobago say how thrilled I have been, that Trinidad has been admitted to full membership of the ICN. Words fail me to say how moved I was when this was announced at the meeting of the Grand Council, and at the spontaneity of the welcome received on that occasion. I have been greatly inspired and stimulated by the scope of the interest and work of the various committees as presented by the Grand Council and I am therefore conscious of the honour conferred on us in being admitted to this fellowship. It is superfluous to say that our profession and our community in Trinidad will benefit from your generosity; but one wonders what can we contribute to this great organization? However, since 'little drops of water, and little grains of sand make the mighty ocean and the pleasant land', I can only promise that we shall try to be worthy of membership, by seeing that in our country we keep pace with the great developments, and by adapting them to the needs of our community.

May I thank most sincerely, the Officers and Staff of Headquarters who have helped us to achieve this membership; and finally the Brazilian Graduate Nurses' Association for their magnificent hospitality and generosity.[12]

As president of the national association, Ben became a member of the board of directors of the ICN. Consequently, she attended international board meetings during her terms of office from 1950 to 1958.[13] Membership opened the whole world of nursing to the association and gave them a global perspective of trends and issues. As Ben observed, "Being on the board meant every document that was passed to board members came here to us. So we were really, very... educated. It was a wonderful form of education for us... It went direct to our members."

The following ICN board meeting was held in Turkey in 1955. Instead of attending it herself, Ben empowered other members to attend as proxies so that they could have the exposure to international events. Evelyn Hargreaves was such a proxy. In 1957 the ICN quadrennial congress was held in Rome, and each national association could send five delegates. The government agreed to assist

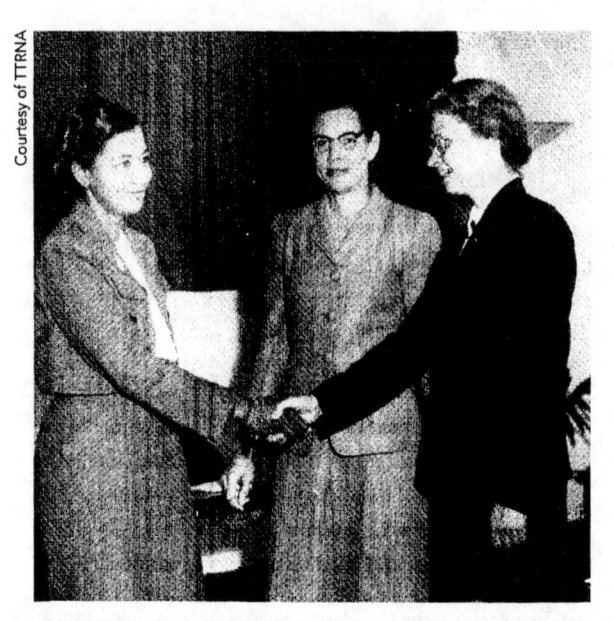

Admission to the International Council of Nurses, Brazil, 1953. At left, Ben shaking hands with Gerda Hoyer, the president of International Council of Nurses, while Thelma Evelyn, the representative for Jamaica, looks on

with the cost for the official delegates, that is, for Ben as the president, and for the secretary. Always thinking of the professional development of her colleagues, Ben suggested to the executive that instead of using the money for the two of them, it be shared equally so that five delegates could attend, with all contributing part of the expenses. This strategy met with the approval of the government and made it possible for five delegates, Ben, Ivy Darmanie, Grace Bayley, Irene Montenegro and Pearl Peters, to attend the congress.

Membership in ICN exposed the local nurses to advances in nursing service and education and the problems of nursing worldwide. Ben declared, "It was a wonderful opening for the profession here. And we have participated regularly. From time to time we had visitors from there come down. Or if nurses were going on study leave . . . they could get facilities abroad, get exchange programmes." For Ben, it was not merely her efforts but, "there was a core, a hard core of nurses who worked extremely hard." Some of them were nurses whom she met in the association and among them was one of the founders of the Southern Certificated Nurses' Association, Miss Irene Montenegro. At the fiftieth anniversary celebra-

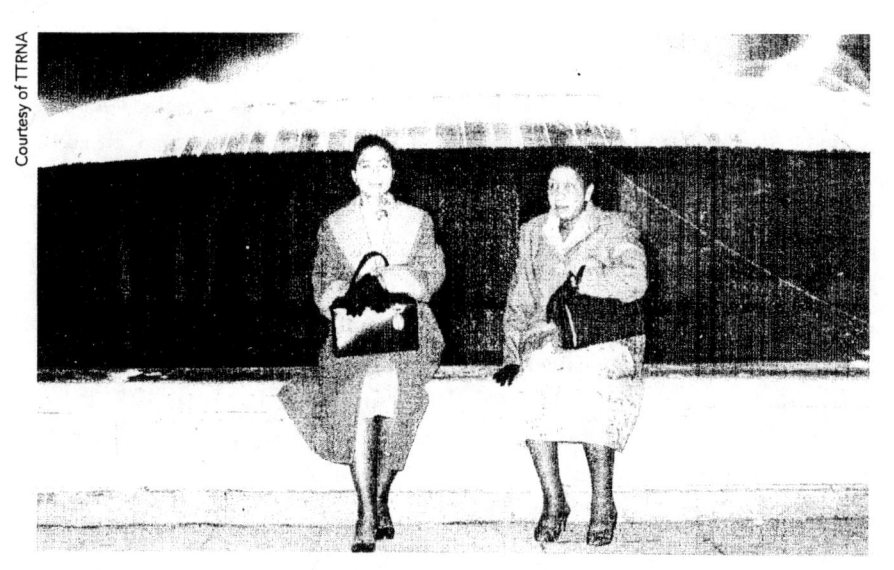

Ben sightseeing with Pearl Peters, International Council of Nurses' congress, Rome, 1957

tion of the TTRNA in 1980, Irene Montenegro, former junior matron of the San Fernando Hospital, paid tribute to Ben in her "Random Jottings from the Early Days":

> I cannot allow this 50th anniversary to pass without paying tribute to one of our most outstanding members who became Secretary shortly after she qualified in nursing and midwifery in 1940/41 and is still in harness today.
>
> I claim the privilege of having invigilated her test paper for admission to hospital. Matron Bridget Ristori, a Florence Nightingale National Nursing Fellow, admitted her to begin her studies which she completed in the required time, with the added distinction of winning the Princess Margaret Silver Medal.
>
> She has represented the Association at several overseas conferences (in Great Britain, Brazil, Italy, and the Caribbean Islands) mainly at her husband's expense; she has given valuable time to the affairs of her sister-nurses despite the calls of her family duties as wife and mother of three.
>
> Fellow members, I think we owe an enormous debt of gratitude to our dedicated honorary Executive Secretary, Mrs Berenice Dolly, and her equally selfless husband, Dr Reynold Cartwright Dolly. May God bless them for the many sacrifices they have made throughout their lives for others.[14]

The 1950s were years of consolidation for the nursing profession with Ben continuing at the helm as president of the association from 1950 to 1958.[15] The association during Ben's tenure started refresher courses that were conducted annually. Not content to focus only on the continuing education needs of members, they offered pre-nursing scholarships to enable girls to bridge the gap between leaving school at sixteen and entering training at eighteen, a period when girls of the desired standards of education and suitability were lost to other professions.

During that decade, there was great difficulty in obtaining qualified sister tutors from Britain in adequate numbers or for long periods, and insufficient scholarships were available for tutor training abroad. Those who could afford it pursued training abroad. However, this practice did not benefit the country because many did not return when they had completed their nursing studies. To compound the situation, because of the shortage of nurses in Britain both during and after World War II, the General Nursing Council's entrance examinations in Britain were abolished which led to an open door, since many locally trained nurses could now find posts easily in Britain. The Colonial Office established a selections committee in the Department of Health to facilitate pre-selection and interviewing of candidates who wanted to go to Britain for training. This caused a further drain on local human resources. Ben and Ivy were appointed to that selections committee and it provided them with useful knowledge that they would use in the years ahead to enrich the education of local nurses.

Though the country achieved self-government in 1956, health service staff and the public remained dissatisfied when the unsatisfactory conditions in the health services apparent in the colonial era persisted. In March 1957 the government appointed a commission of enquiry (better known as the Julien Commission) with the following terms of reference: "To survey Hospital facilities in the Colony, to examine the causes and consequences of dissatisfaction with conditions obtaining at government Hospitals, among doctors, nurses, and all grades of staff, particularly among the general public, and to propose remedies and make recommendations for improvement in respect of these matters."[16]

Ben was appointed to this prestigious commission which was both thorough and exhaustive in its deliberations. Forty-seven meetings were held across the nation and visits were conducted to the three colonial hospitals, the several district hospitals, health centres, and clinics throughout Trinidad and Tobago. The commission commented in general on the problem of shortages, particularly as they related to nurses and their training. A high rate of failure in the nurses' preliminary school examination was attributed to the scarcity of qualified sister tutors, and the inability of ward sisters to find sufficient time to teach student nurses because of the serious overcrowding on the wards and the acute shortage of staff. The recommendations of the commission relative to nurses were far-reaching, extending from the selection of candidates to their education, training and conditions of service.

A major thrust spearheaded by the professional association under Ben's leadership was to have locally qualified nurses trained as sister tutors. Few local nurses had been sent to Britain for training, and the reason usually given was that, in general, they did not have the required educational preparation for entry into sister tutor courses. Ben observed, "It was difficult to get qualified tutors to come out and it was difficult to get our nurses accepted for tutor training. And we couldn't understand why." Undaunted, Ben set out to solve this problem. Through her contacts with the General Nursing Council in England, she was told that they would be prepared to send her the requirements, and the entrance test under confidential cover, if she would guarantee the conducting and supervision of the test. Since Ben was not a government service employee, she wisely sought the consent of the director of medical services, Dr Peat, and the cooperation of the schools of nursing. All was approved and the first test was carried out in an office in Port of Spain. This procedure continued for some time until the first tutors were sent abroad through that programme. Those who had successfully completed the test in the island could no longer be rejected.

Simultaneously, the association started courses with the Extra-Mural Department of UWI. The Public Relations Committee was formed, with a representative from the university, community representation, and members of TTRNA, with the goal of introducing science courses in both the north and south of the island. Trinidad, as late as the 1960s, suffered from a lack of science subjects in secondary schools for girls. The programme was conducted for a few years until, as secondary education improved, it was no longer necessary. Ben summed up, "There was some of that [educational preparation] but it was not adequate, so we fought this and had special courses run by the Association with the Extra-Mural Department of the University of the West Indies for tutors . . . I myself went to the Royal College of Nursing in Britain and requested them to send the tests here, and that I would supervise them rather than have nurses go all the way to Britain and perhaps not qualify."

Some of the first tutors came out of this upgrading programme which facilitated their entry into postgraduate programmes abroad. Lucy Fields and Valerie Foster were among the first early nurses who took that test. In 1954 Lucy Fields was the first Trinidad trained nurse to be sent to the United Kingdom on a government scholarship to take the sister tutor's course at the University of Edinburgh; and in

1955 she was subsequently appointed to the position of senior sister tutor, the first Trinidad trained nurse to hold such a position at the colonial hospital in Port of Spain. In this position, Lucy (an ardent advocate for the founding of the Nursing Council) introduced a new dimension to nursing education, based on her experience in Edinburgh, assisting the Nursing Council to give public health and hygiene a prominent place in the syllabus and examinations. Valerie Foster likewise went abroad and on her return held several senior positions. She was a tutor, director of the School of Nursing in Port of Spain and, subsequently, principal nursing officer for Trinidad and Tobago until her retirement in the late eighties.[17]

BEN'S INFLUENCE ON THE REGION

Towards the end of Ben's term of office in 1958, nurses in the West Indies were taking action to encourage regional cooperation. The period from 1958 to 1961 saw the newly formed Federation of the West Indies come into being and this facilitated cooperation of both a governmental and nongovernmental nature in nursing. Nurses in the West Indies had felt the need for regional cooperation for a long time and successive reports during the colonial era had advised such a development. While there had been interisland communication from time to time, as exemplified by Trinidadian, Jamaican and Guyanese nurses regarding registration, it was not until 1957 that a group of nurses in Antigua, headed by Mavis Harney-Brown, called a conference to inaugurate the CNO. The main objective was to assist the territories to achieve some common acceptable standards of education for nurses. The organization encompassed not only the British territories but also the French and Dutch West Indies, Puerto Rico and the American Virgin Islands, and proposed biennial meetings in different member countries. Membership was of two types: group membership through territorial professional association, or individual membership. Ben was the TTRNA president when the inaugural meeting of the CNO was held in Antigua but the Trinidad and Tobago delegation was unable to attend. They were already committed to attend, for the first time since their association's admission to the ICN, the international nursing congress in Rome. However, one of the active members of the TTRNA, Veronica Awon, attended. TTRNA was admitted to CNO in 1959 and has participated fully in all its activities since. There was no obligation for the association of any particular territory to join, but all have done so. The CNO has remained a valuable

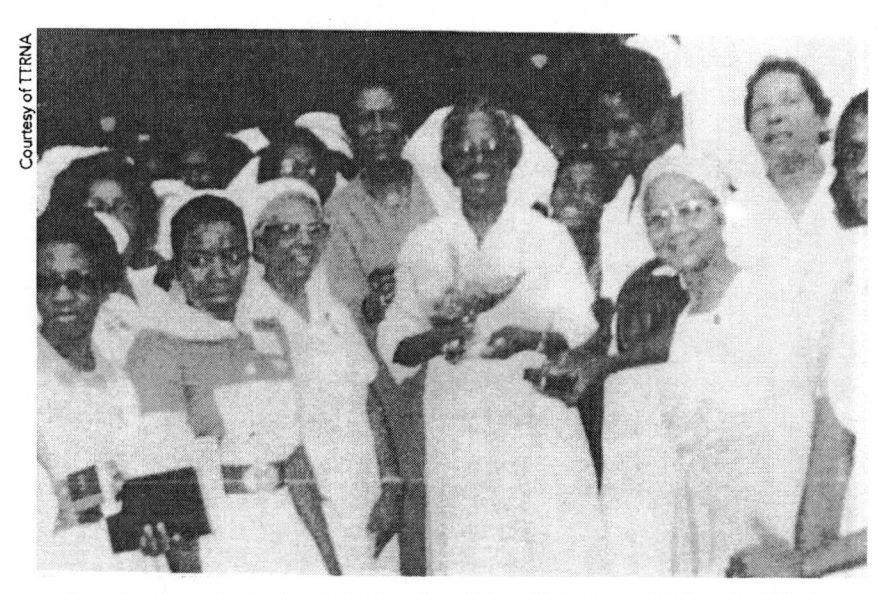

At front, far right, Ben with Laurel McDowell, president of Trinidad and Tobago Registered Nurses' Association, and Caribbean nurses after church service, Caribbean Nurses' Organization biennial conference, Trinidad, 1980

means of nongovernmental coordination, cooperation, encouragement, and stimulation for the benefit of Caribbean nursing education and health care.

Although Ben was never an officer of the organization, she responded whenever called upon to assist with constitutional matters. It was recognized that she had considerable experience through her intimate involvement with TTRNA nursing registration law, though she herself downplays her contribution, commenting, "In my public life I have had a lot of exposure to legal work. I worked on the law of the Attorney General's Commission . . . I have been fortunate to have acquired that knowledge. So I usually function at these conferences in that role apart from being a full participant, of course . . . I would not consider that my contribution to CNO is greater than any other active member's should be." Ben's legal knowledge has been acknowledged by others. Yvonne Pilgrim, current executive secretary of TTRNA, observed, "She has a very keen, legal mind and would see the legal implications in many situations."[18]

On 31 August 1959 a group of senior nursing personnel (sponsored and selected by their governments) from the Commonwealth Caribbean came together in Barbados, for the first time in the history of nursing in the Caribbean, to discuss the problems confronting them. Ben Dolly attended as the representative for the

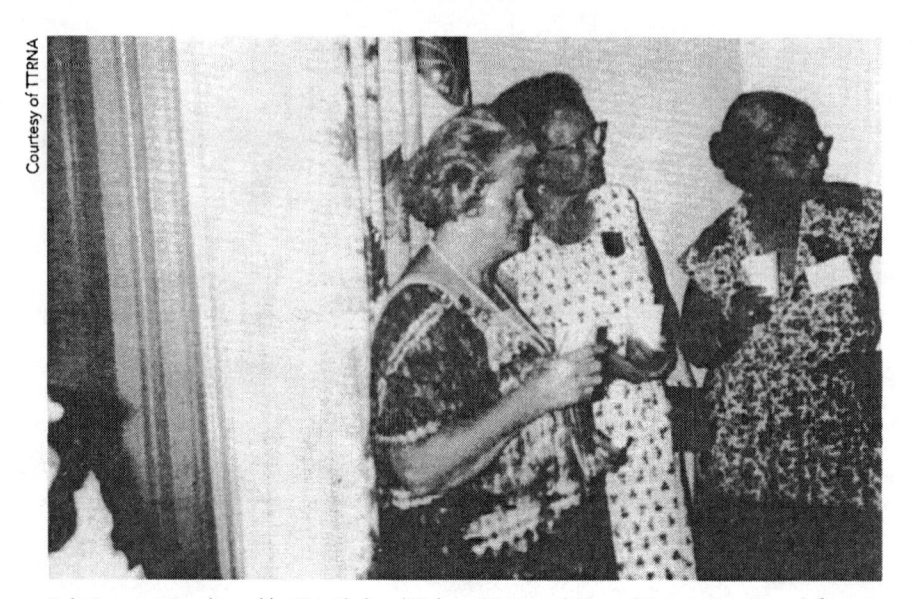

Relaxing at a party hosted by Trinidad and Tobago Registered Nurses' Association. From left to right, Margaret Brayton, (executive secretary, Commonwealth Nurses' Foundation), Anna Stanislaus, and Ben at the thirteenth biennial conference, Caribbean Nurses' Organization, Bahamas, 1982

Nursing Council of Trinidad and Tobago. It was a historic conference held under the auspices of the newly formed Federal Government of the West Indies and chaired by Dr Horace Gillette, federal medical advisor. Evolving from this conference was a steering committee comprised of eight members. They were Berenice Dolly, General Nursing Council, Trinidad; Eunice Baber, matron of the Belize City Hospital, British Honduras; R. Clapton, principal matron, Medical Department, Nassau, Bahamas (though she discontinued as a member of the Board of Review before the completion of the survey); Monica Clyne, nursing superintendent, Medical Department, St George's, Grenada; Marion Harding, matron, Georgetown Hospital, British Guiana; Eva Lowe, acting principal officer, Ministry of Health, Jamaica; May Stevens, matron, Cunningham Hospital, St Kitts; and Ena Walters, matron, Queen Elizabeth Hospital, Barbados. One of the tasks of the committee was to carry out a thorough review of the recommendations of the conference. Ben was nominated by one of the island representatives to be the secretary of this steering committee, which met in Trinidad in 1961 to carry out its task as envisioned by the conference. In 1963 the plan of the steering committee was submitted to PAHO/WHO. The committee had recommended a survey of the schools of nursing in the region and members subsequently served on the advisory committee which Nita Barrow headed. It became a board of review for the evaluation of the schools of nursing in the thirteen territories.[19] Ben thus became involved in evaluating schools in the region.

Counsellor and Advisor

Although the presidency of TTRNA was subsequently assumed by others, Ben would continue to play a pivotal role in nursing and community affairs. In 1963 she was again elected president and remained in office until 1967. The experience of Ben and of Ivy Waterman on the Department of Health Selections Committee for many years during the forties made them aware that many nurses experienced difficulty in being accepted in post-diploma programmes in Great Britain. They identified the issue as a lack of knowledge of the basic procedure of applying, knowledge about the programme and conditions abroad, among others. Consequently, in 1964 the association, under Ben's leadership, formed a counselling programme called the Trinidad Counselling and Advisory Service (TRINCAS) with the intent of operating at two levels. On one level, it advised prospective students for training in the island and abroad, encouraged good students to train locally to forestall the need to recruit foreign nurses, and advised on cultural factors to assist in adaptation abroad. Ben noted, "Because of our historical past, it was assumed that any hospital in the United Kingdom was better than the hospitals here. We [those of us who had travelled] knew that was not a fact, and therefore tried to guide them into the type of hospital that would be suitable for the applicant."

The procedure required students to apply to the association's office, and pay a small fee, and TRINCAS would contact the hospitals on their behalf, and make

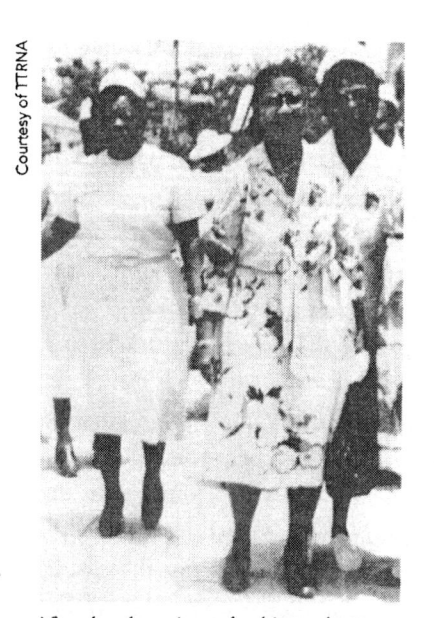

After church service at the thirteenth biennial conference, Caribbean Nurses' Organization, Bahamas, 1982. At centre, Ben Dolly, with Yvonne Pilgrim, executive secretary, on the right and A. Stanislaus on the left

the telephone calls for which, if they were long distance, the candidate would pay the costs. While TRINCAS was not an official selection process, Ben acknowledged that the hospitals in the United Kingdom accepted persons sent by them, and the service was perceived unofficially as a pre-selection process. It was a fruitful exercise: the hospitals in Great Britain were pleased that a nursing organization was doing a pre-selection, as they were at a disadvantage in making judgments and "were sometimes misjudged as to the reasons why they rejected applicants". This service ultimately benefited both the local candidates and the hospitals. Though some of these candidates did settle abroad after their studies, many of them returned to Trinidad and Tobago to work.

At the second level, TRINCAS also assisted graduate nurses who wanted to do post-basic work by helping to guide them to the type of hospital that would be most appropriate for them or would provide richer experience than that available in the island. The Royal College of Nursing was very helpful in this venture. Information about hospitals gained from the International Exchange Programme of the ICN, coupled with the knowledge about nursing legislation garnered through experience in the Nursing Council, assisted TRINCAS in guiding registered nurses in making wise choices and adjusting to their new environment.

It was indeed a busy and rewarding time for the association and its services. The success of this endeavour, long since ended when circumstances changed and the service was no longer needed, is seen in recent times as many nurses who benefited from that service still keep in contact with Ben. She recounted, "They would say, 'Mrs Dolly, you don't remember me? And I say, 'What is your name?' They would say, 'You sent me to do nursing.' That is how they would put it: 'You sent me to do nursing.' Well, as soon as they would say that I would know that it was through the association programme." Colleen Alexander (Joseph) was one such recipient. She returned to Trinidad to work as a staff nurse at the Mount Hope Maternity Hospital after twelve years abroad where she qualified as a registered nurse, a certified midwife, a registered mental nurse and became a ward sister.

Ben was most helpful in guiding nurses in the mechanics of completing application forms. While this may seem trivial, its importance cannot be underestimated. Understanding the terminology on overseas application forms and getting them completed in time can at times be difficult. Ben pointed out, "One of the things we learned from international membership (in ICN) is the very important fact of learning the international language. People will apply on a foreign form and use terms . . . which only mean something locally."

During the period of grave shortage of trained nurses, the government was seeking to recruit local nurses once they had qualified in Britain. Ben had many contacts through the ICN when she was a board member, and on one of her trips to England, the office of the matron of the Middlesex Hospital was at her disposal to conduct interviews for nurses for recruitment to Trinidad. Because Ben was not there as an official representative of the government but in a private capacity or as an association executive, she declined the offer. However, she spoke at association meetings in England and to individuals, encouraging them to return to Trinidad, as well as guiding them to take courses that would be of value for work in the island. Midwifery tutors were sorely needed, so nurse recruits were encouraged to pursue midwifery programmes. Ben, true to character, was not satisfied merely to advise them; she wanted to be knowledgeable about such programmes. She went to the Central Midwives Board to get the necessary information so that she could share it wisely with those she encountered or sought out. She said, "I have always been convinced that if I was asked to do anything, any form of service, and I had the opportunity to try to do it, that I should do it . . . and in many cases I was better placed to do it. Because one of the reasons why I was able to do some things was the fact that I was not a government employee . . . I was able to speak out as an independent voice. That was the main reason really . . . During all those years, it was important to nursing to be able to have somebody speak who was not subject to the conditions of service that they might have been subject to politically as well as otherwise."

The Path to Professional Development

Always propelled by a desire to improve her knowledge base, Ben went to the University of Edinburgh for post-basic studies in nursing administration in 1965. The Department of Nursing Studies had two programmes. One was the International School in which students from all over the world took courses in either the nurse tutor programme or nursing administration. The WHO showed interest by supporting WHO fellows to enrol in those programmes. Most, if not all, students in the international programme were funded by WHO or their governments, but not Ben. She was not a government employee and, as such, could not be sponsored. Ben studied economics as an elective as she felt that it was an area of expertise lacking in nurses in the island. Ben was somewhat concerned as to whether she would be accepted into the programme since she was "removed from bedside nursing", but in her interview, she was told, "Mrs Dolly if you have done all that you have done, as well as raised a family, you're more than qualified to enter the department. You should be coming here to teach." Her studies were an enriching experience. Like Nita Barrow who was not so interested in getting a degree or qualifications per se but as self-development, Ben said, "I was not interested only in the question of getting the qualification as such . . . I had been going from one level to the other here . . . I mean growing, developing . . . Even though you are doing activities in the interest of something else, you grow and develop as well." Her programme of studies, where she encountered nurses from Africa, Greece, Poland and other parts of the world, exposed her to seeing and experiencing the administrative, public health and the curative aspects of health care. It was, in her words, "a wonderful experience". It was here that she met Dr Margaret Scott Wright, a brilliant nurse, who later became the first holder of the newly established chair of nursing studies at the University of Edinburgh, the first chair of nursing in Europe.

International Experiences

From as early as the 1950s to the late 1970s, Ben was frequently Trinidad's representative for the League of Women Voters (which was affiliated to the British Commonwealth League in Britain), the Soroptimists International, the International Alliance of Women, and similar voluntary agencies at meetings internationally. Further, she always seized the opportunity while on trips to Britain with her husband to advocate for nursing in Trinidad with the General Nursing Council, the Royal College of Nursing and other nursing organizations. She gained further international exposure during her term as a member of the board of directors of the ICN when she was president of the nurses' association from the late 1940s to the late 1950s.

In 1966 Ben's recognition of the importance of international linkages led her to assist in the formation of the Commonwealth Nurses' Federation in Montreal, Canada, on the occasion of the ICN quadrennial congress. Margaret Brayton was the executive director of the Commonwealth Federation based in Britain and she and Ben seized the opportunity to form the Commonwealth Nurses' Federation, which has subsequently used these international or regional meetings of ICN to 'piggyback' and host federation meetings. These activities provided valuable learning experiences not only for Ben but for nursing in Trinidad and Tobago.

Valerie Alleyne Rawlins, quality care manager, Ministry of Health, captured this notion well in her recent tribute to Ben, in 1997, on the occasion of her eightieth birthday when she was honoured for her contributions to nursing by the southern branch of the TTRNA:

> I am sure that it is no coincidence that every time Mrs Dolly expanded her knowledge base or benefited from some learning experience, there was some concomitant development or innovation at the professional association . . . An activist with great professional acumen, she always advocated the need for nurses to view nursing in a global context – to quote her own words 'against the backdrop of the world' – since insularity could only impede the growth of the profession.[20]

EXECUTIVE SECRETARY OF TTRNA

After those decades of service, Ben was appointed TTRNA executive secretary in 1967 when the constitution was changed to allow a staff position. The intent of the association was to eventually make it a salaried position but that was never realized and it remains a voluntary position. This has created some problems as it inevitably meant that the nurse in the staff position has full-time employment elsewhere and has to burn the midnight oil regularly in order to carry out their duties. Ben observed regretfully that the full extent of the job is not fully appreciated by membership and that it is taken for granted. She elaborated on this point, "In fact, it is really looked upon as a position of privilege, rather than what it is. Just a drudge, hard work position, in which everything is on your back and you have the responsibility for everything. But it is difficult in a country like this to have the number of people who would be willing to accept that position, and who would do it efficiently."

Yvonne Pilgrim, former principal of the School of Nursing, San Fernando, has held that position since Ben retired in 1980 because of failing health. She described how she learned from Ben by "understudying" her from 1977. Yvonne assumed the responsibility for carrying out all the functions with Ben still in the official role before she was formally nominated to the position in 1981.

Ben proudly said that while she was the executive secretary in 1977, Jean Grayson (now Dr Grayson) had been nominated by the association to the ICN for the 3M International Award and was the first nurse from the island to win this prestigious international award. It enabled her to do her master's degree in nursing at Boston University. Ben contended that the depth of the nursing education of local nurses was underestimated. This belief was grounded in her own experience in Scotland. While taking her post-basic studies there, she was continually asked why she had not applied for a master's programme as she was studying with some people who did not have her depth of knowledge or experience. She insisted, "and so I may have said this to you before, and I repeat it, that while the post-basic courses the nurses went for expanded their knowledge in a lateral way, they never went to a higher level. They were never exposed to a higher level of nursing education. And so, in a way, their abilities were wasted in the time of study abroad. They themselves did not appreciate what they were worth and I think that kept us back for a number of years."

Forever a mentor, she advised Jean, who was a nurse tutor with several years of experience, to apply for the master's programme at Boston University. While it appeared inconceivable at that time that one could apply for a master's degree without a bachelor's degree, Jean did, and was admitted on the basis of her knowledge and experience. There were a few courses that she was required to take at the bachelor's level, but Ben's point was well taken. Jean, who recently retired as principal nursing officer, credited Ben with encouraging her to apply for the 3M International Fellowship and for suggesting that she aspire for the master's degree. Jean was glowing in her praise of Ben's contributions, "I, in a way, see her as my mentor, certainly because I got a tremendous amount of encouragement from her. She encouraged me every step of the way . . . as a member of the northern branch and a member of the central executive of the Association . . . for the 3M fellowship . . . She said that we as nurses didn't see our own capabilities . . . She used Nita Barrow as an example . . . Why settle just for the bachelor's degree? . . . Seek to find out whether there was something else possible, like a master's degree."[21] Jean elaborated on Ben's qualities and accomplishments. Her words echo the views of many: "I think that Mrs Dolly has been and is one of our most prestigious nursing leaders. She has been, I think, a mentor to many, many nurses, especially those who belong to the nursing association in Trinidad and Tobago. Because she has advised nurses. She has quietly identified those whom she thought would ensure the progress of the association. She tried to help those persons in terms of providing advice and pointing them in a certain direction. Mrs Dolly, I would call her in a way, an academic sort of person. Although she is very practical too . . . because of her background in the association and in education and development, brought something that was different to nursing, at that time. She was the one who saw the potential in people and in the nursing organization."

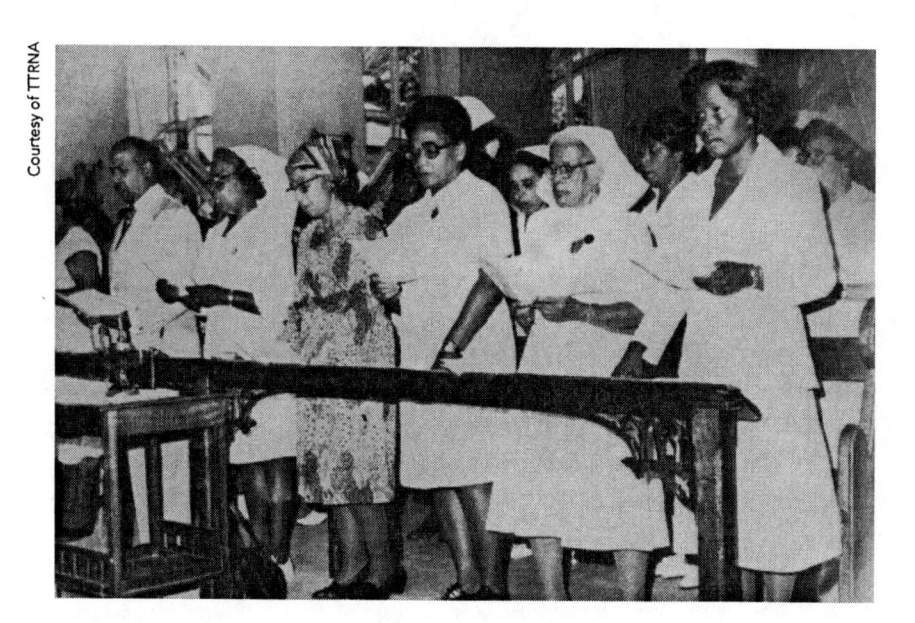

Ben participating in the church service, Nurses' Week 1979. From left to right, Sir Ellis Clarke (president of the Republic of Trinidad and Tobago), Laurel McDowell, Ben Dolly, Evelyn Hargreaves, Irene Mitchell, and Angela Bacchus

Ben's contribution to many nurses was "the opening of doors and the opening of the eyes of nurses to the fact that they were worth much more than they were seeing themselves as". This vital insight was most useful to local nurses as it raised their self-esteem to a level that, in pursuit of advanced studies, they were no longer hesitant to aspire to higher levels. In fact, the official government-sponsored scholarships were eventually offered at a more advanced level, that is, for a master's degree at universities abroad. In 1980, when the TTRNA celebrated their fiftieth anniversary, for the first time in the history of the association the decision was made to issue awards to members for their service. In a long overdue ceremony, Ben received their distinguished service award that year.

Like their counterparts in Jamaica, the nurses had a lot of difficulty in acquiring land to build their headquarters due to lack of financial resources. The Commonwealth Foundation in Britain established a project in the 1960s to set up professional centres throughout the Commonwealth. The objectives were to bring professionals together to be a force in the community on matters of importance and also to bring the professions closer together so they could interact better for the good of the community. Because of its international connections and communications with the office in Britain, the association was aware of the impending visit to Trinidad in 1968 by Mr Chadwick who represented the foundation. The executive made certain that an interview with him would be arranged. Following the visit, Trinidad and Tobago was one of the countries that received a grant towards the setting up of such a centre. Eventually, land was allocated by the public authorities branch of the government and a headquarters was built. The building, named the Professional Centre, was erected with funds from the professional bodies currently housed there and opened in December 1985. The TTRNA acquired a board room, a small office, library and kitchen. Other organizations housed in the centre are the associations of chartered accountants, professional engineers and pharmacists.

Although the accommodation is not entirely what was hoped for, the association at long last has its headquarters. Ben said, "I am very happy that we did that achievement because it has helped us a lot. Part of the reason why we can't find all of our records is the fact that they had to be at my house sometimes and they had to be at somebody else's house sometimes!"

In 1984 Ben travelled to New York where she was honoured with an award by the Trinidad and Tobago Alliance of the United States of America Incorporated, as a pioneer in the field of nursing. Finally, in 1991, at the Third Quadrennial Health Conference co-sponsored by nurses of TTRNA and the Trinidad and Tobago Nurses' Association of America, a tribute was paid to Ben by TTRNA for outstanding service to the nursing profession and the people of the twin island state. Ben echoed Dame Nita's sentiments and modesty when she insisted that these achievements and honours were not hers but those of "so many support people, so many loyal people . . . You are elected by them and placed in the position and it's truly a support, really, that you're able to remain a leader. I think I owe a lot of it to people who have been so loyal, conscientious. I think that we can feel happy about certain things."

Jean Grayson corroborated the point of view held by many about Ben's integrity and elaborated: "She is a very, very honest person. She has a great deal of integrity and sticks to principles. Caring. I don't think people always saw that side and sometimes misunderstood the integrity and the principal action. The loyalty, loyal to people to a fault, perhaps. In terms of economic well-being for our nurses; perhaps this was not as high on her agenda. Perhaps it ought to be, but it was not neglected either . . . If there was one particular goal, it was that nursing should function as any other major discipline and be recognized as such by the people of Trinidad and Tobago . . . When I was chief nursing officer and we had delegations

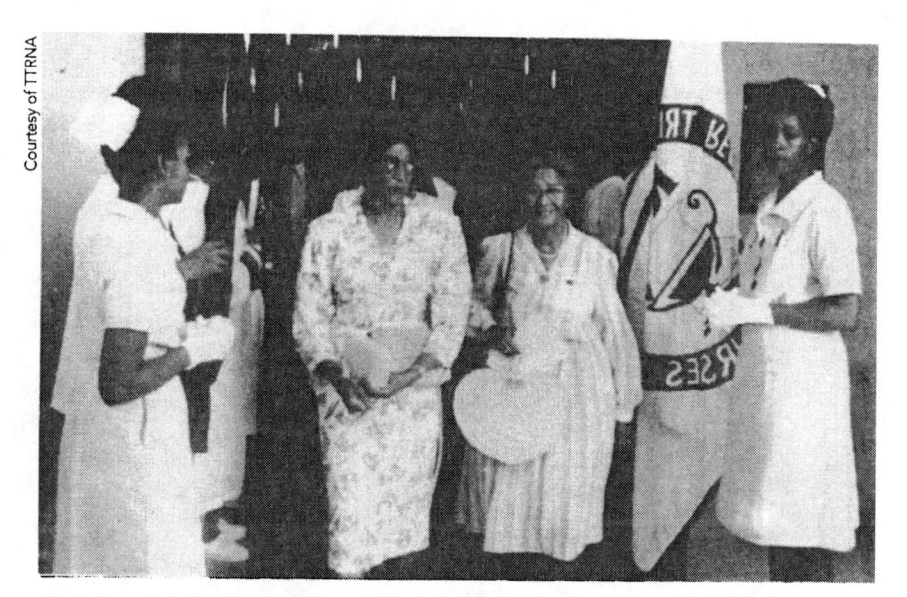

Second quadrennial health seminar, 1987. Ben and Mrs Hassanali, wife of the president of the Republic of Trinidad and Tobago, leaving the church service

from the association or the Nursing Council, if Mrs Dolly was a member of the delegation, one would observe how the minister [of health] and the permanent secretary and others listened intently to what she had to say with respect to what had been done in the past, and what was required and what we [nurses] would be prepared to give towards the country. They had great respect and regard for her and what she has done, not only for nursing but for health generally."

Ben reiterated the risks that local nurses such as Irene Montenegro and Irene Mitchell took, against all odds, in the early years to get conditions changed for nursing, and she considered them leaders and stalwarts of nursing. But to Yvonne Pilgrim, Valerie Rawlins, Dr Jean Grayson and many others, Ben herself was a mentor par excellence. Yvonne characterized her as one who "had the ability to recognize abilities in others and motivate them to go forward and assist them whenever possible".[22] She lavished praise on Ben: "I think she is an excellent leader. Where the leader does not feel threatened, they are so assured in self and abilities that they can recognize the abilities in others and not feel threatened. And promote them for the welfare of the profession and the good of the country. So I have no hesitation in saying that she is an excellent leader . . . She has always advocated

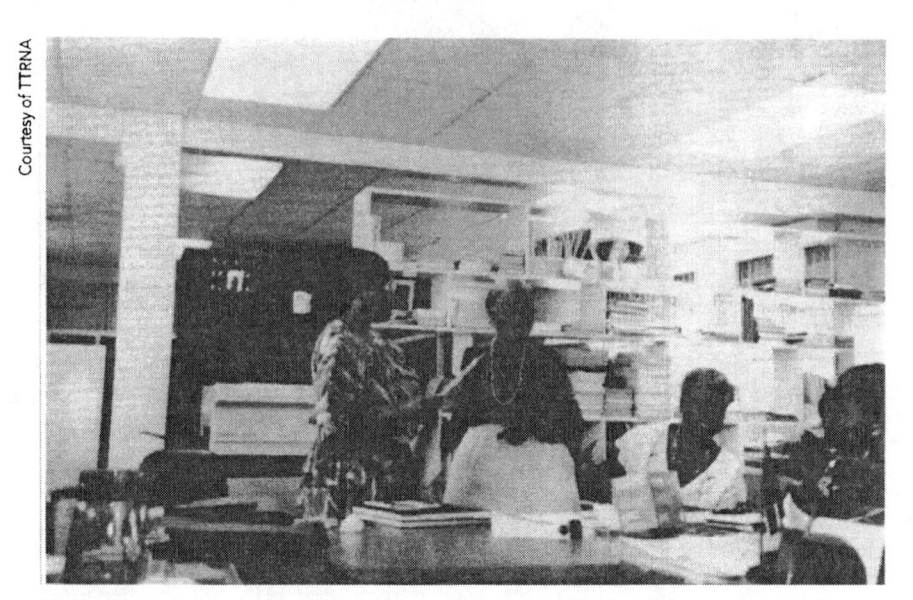

Working behind the scenes at the biennial general meeting, 1994. From left to right, B. Parris, Ben Dolly, I. Gilbert, A. Nelson, and Yvonne Pilgrim

strongly for the community and welcomed the present shift in focus that is the basis of all health sector reform, primary health care."

Ben believed that there were present-day nurses who were carrying the torch forward but worried about the future graduates from the 'new' nursing programme at NIHERST, whether they would become involved in more than their jobs. "We have to work at getting them involved in professionalism, in the wider sense. That will be the key to it." And that, indeed, was the key to Ben's commitment for, at seventy-nine, she was able to say that nursing "is something you enter and have a responsibility to develop all your life". It is a telling and lasting tribute to her when Yvonne commented that "this outstanding nurse continues to ensure that the commitment made in 1953 to the ICN is still being upheld through the guidance and counselling she gives to all". That view was further validated by Valerie Alleyne Rawlins:

Many can attest to the fact that her love for nursing and concern for humanity motivated all her actions. It is said that effective nurse leaders are visionaries, facilitators, risk-takers, decision-makers, activists, and exceptional role models, persons who believe and behave as though they have the responsibility to role-model all expected actions and words all of the time. A role model she has been, and continues to be.[23]

In his book *The Seven Habits of Highly Effective People,* Steven Covey observes that integrity includes but goes beyond honesty. Integrity is keeping promises and fulfilling expectations. It requires an integrated character, a oneness, primarily with self but also with life.[24] A woman of integrity and a guiding light for Caribbean nurses and women is Ben Dolly: pioneer, mentor, advocate, leader, wife, mother – and ever a nurse.

NOTES

1. B. Brereton, *A History of Modern Trinidad, 1783–1962* (London: Heinemann, 1981), 122–30; P. Mohammed, "Women and Education", in *Women in the Caribbean Project,* vol. 5, edited by Joycelin Massiah (Cave Hill, Barbados: Institute of Social and Economic Research, 1982), 35–37.
2. R.E. Reddock, *Women, Labour and Struggle in Twentieth Century Trinidad and Tobago, 1898–1960* (The Hague: Institute of Social Studies, 1984), 295–98.
3. I. Waterman, "A Century of Service", *The Nursing Council of Trinidad and Tobago 25th Anniversary, 1950–1975* (Port of Spain, Trinidad: Key Caribbean Publications, 1975), 15.
4. *Trinidad and Tobago Registered Nurses' Association: Fifty Years of Service, 1930–1980* (Port of Spain, Trinidad: Trinidad and Tobago Registered Nurses' Association, c. 1980).
5. This is a system where nursing students had continuous classroom lectures for a given period of time, for example, one or two weeks or months, with clinical practice at the end of that time.
6. *Report of the Committee on the Training of Nurses for the Colonies,* Cmd. 6672 (1945), 9; M. Bryce-Boodoo, "A Fresh Look at Nursing Education in Trinidad and Tobago", *The Nursing Council of Trinidad and Tobago 25th Anniversary, 1950–1975* (Port of Spain, Trinidad: Key Publications, 1975), 33.
7. B. Dolly, "The Development of Nursing Education in Trinidad and Tobago", (typescript, 1966).
8. *Trinidad and Tobago Registered Nurses' Association: Fifty Years of Service,* 19.
9. *The Nursing Council of Trinidad and Tobago 25th Anniversary, 1950–1975,* 8.
10. Pearl Peters, personal interview, February 1996. All material quoted from Peters is from this interview.
11. Lynne Beckles, personal interview, March 1996. All material quoted from Lynne Beckles is from this interview.

12. *Trinidad and Tobago Registered Nurses' Association: Fifty Years of Service*, 14.
13. Because of the large number of countries currently included in ICN membership, the structure has changed, where the president is no longer a member of the board. There is now an executive which carries out the day-to-day and year-to-year activities in between conferences. The presidents sit on the Council of National Representatives (CNR).
14. *Trinidad and Tobago Registered Nurses' Association: Fifty Years of Service*, 33–34.
15. In recent years, a constitutional amendment has limited the presidency to two consecutive terms of two years per term. One can resume office after a break.
16. *Report of the Commission of Enquiry*, M.T. Julien, chairman, Council Paper no. 14 (Port of Spain, Trinidad, 1957), 1, 55.
17. J. Hezekiah, "The Development of Nursing Education: 1956–1986" (PhD diss., University of Alberta, Edmonton, 1987), 95–106, 196–221, where the struggle to attain local leadership is examined and analysed.
18. Yvonne Pilgrim, personal interview, February 1996.
19. See chapter 2, nn. 6, 7, where this conference is discussed in greater detail.
20. Valerie Alleyne Rawlins, citation delivered to the southern branch of the TTRNA, July 1997.
21. Jean Grayson, personal interview, May 1996. All material quoted from Grayson in this chapter is from this interview.
22. Yvonne Pilgrim, personal interview, April 1996. Subsequent quotes from Pilgrim in this chapter are from this interview.
23. Rawlins, citation.
24. S.R. Covey, *The Seven Habits of Highly Effective People* (New York: Simon and Schuster, 1990), 195–96.

PART III

Mary Jane Seivwright

Stands must be taken. If I am to respect myself, I have to search myself for what I believe is right and take a stand on what I find. Otherwise I have not gathered together what I have been given, I have not embraced what I have learned: I lack my own conviction.

Hugh Prather

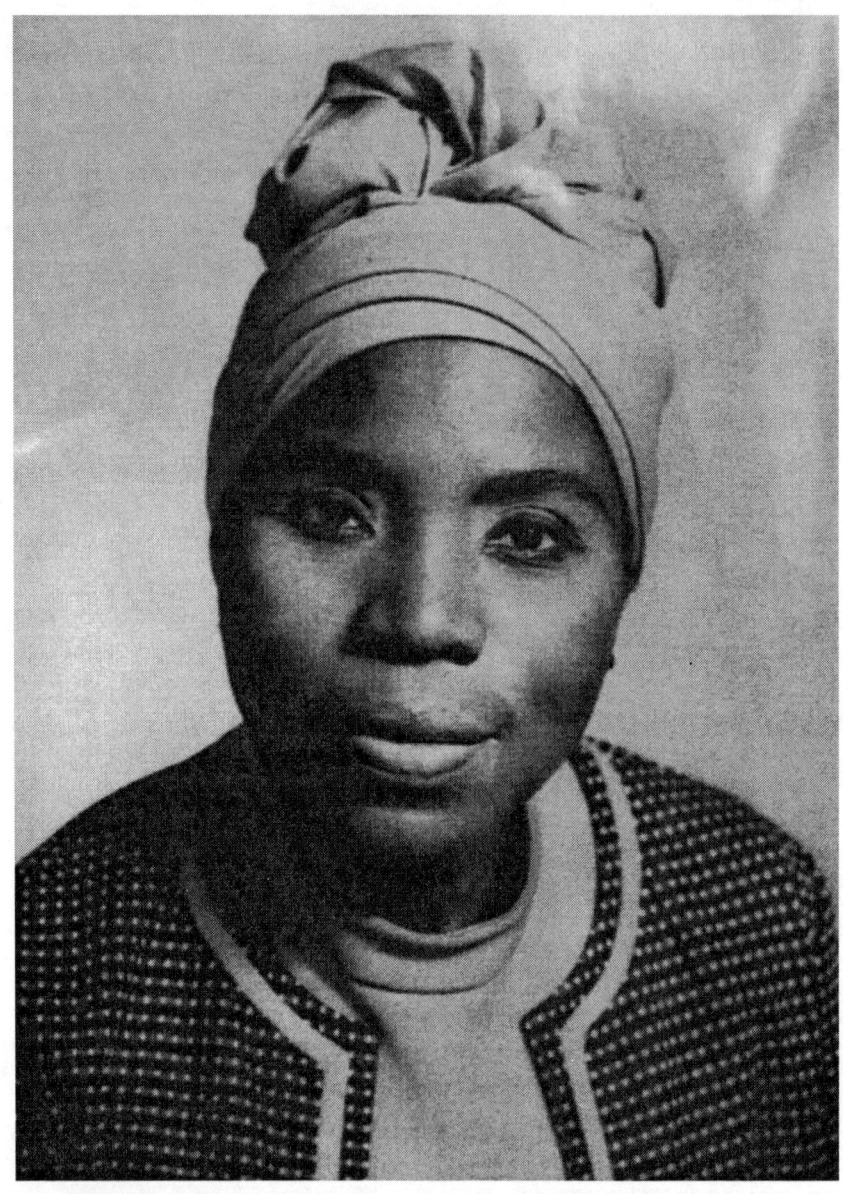

Mary Jane Seivwright, president of the Nurses' Association of Jamaica (1974, 1975, 1980)

CHAPTER FIVE

Beating the Odds

I met Mary Jane Seivwright in many parts of the world on many occasions, all connected with nursing. The venue might be a congress or conferences of the ICN or the CNO, but the one that stands out most was at the Department of Advanced Nursing Annual Nursing Research Conference and Mary Jane Seivwright Day at UWI, Mona, Jamaica, in April 1993. The conference is an annual celebration of Mary's major contribution to nursing in general, and to nursing research, particularly in Jamaica and the Caribbean. Even though she was incapacitated by recent surgery, Mary attended the event in a wheelchair. Her fortitude and determination to be there for present and aspiring students and faculty nurse researchers took precedence over her physical condition. Selfless devotion to research in nursing is the hallmark of this woman.

Mary Jane Seivwright was born on 12 April 1923, the middle of three daughters born to Richard and Martha Seivwright in the small village of Endeavour in Gibraltar, in the parish of St Ann, Jamaica. Mary's older sister married and had two sons, who now live in England, and her younger sister also married and had twelve children, of whom ten survived. It was difficult for her younger sister to support such a large family so Mary 'adopted' the two eldest girls, not in the legal but in the symbolic sense of the word, in that she supported them financially and otherwise. This arrangement is not unusual in the West Indies where it often happens that an aunt or a family member who is financially more secure cares for one or more children of a close relative. As she remarked, in the local parlance, "I took the two girls away and I mind them . . . Such lovely children." She sent them to private secondary schools and paid for their board and lodgings in Kingston where they lived with someone from their same neighbourhood, Gibraltar, who had set up a boarding centre in Kingston for young people from the rural areas. Mary speaks highly of both of them and that they are her surrogate children is without a doubt. She regards them as such and "people regard them as my children; I am very close to them". She was determined to give them an education because "God made me be the first girl to leave my district for a profession, as all got pregnant." The implied message was that she made sure to create a similar opportunity for them as she had for herself. Education then, as it is now, is the key to moving out of poverty into the middle class.

She told me that both nieces now have master's degrees. One is a nurse practitioner and the other is a social worker. They are both married, have their own families and live in the United States. With much affection in her voice, Mary said that they never forget her birthday or Christmas and send her cheques on those occasions. Likewise, her older sister's two sons who live in London also send cheques to her at Christmas. To understand this remarkable woman and to realize how phenomenal her success has been, it is necessary to see her against the background she grew up in and the conditions of the time.

The Landscape of Her Birth

Jamaica, a mountainous island of about 4,441 square miles with a population of 2,500,000, remained in continuous English occupation from the time of its capture by the British in 1655 until independence in 1962. St Ann, known as the Garden Parish of Jamaica, is primarily agricultural, with bananas, pimento, sugarcane, coconuts, coffee, citrus and sisal as the main crops. Mary's parents were poor and had to eke out a living for themselves. Her father was a small-scale subsistence farmer and her mother remained at home to care for the family. The historical significance of small-scale, private agricultural cultivation and landholding in rural areas, which were 98 percent black, is that it is a legacy of the Jamaican working class, linked to the legacy of slavery. There was a self-respecting peasantry of small landholders who raised their own food crops on their own farms and supplemented their own production with wage labour on plantations when desirable. The importance of landholding in the postemancipation period was central in the ideology of the peasantry. It became a pivotal issue in class conflict in the Morant Bay uprising of 1865 which led to political changes. By 1900 new ideas about civil, political, economic and social equality were spreading. The financial qualification of voters had been reduced by 1919 and there was female suffrage on a restricted basis.

In the 1920s the composition of the Legislative Council had so changed that, among the elected members, the blacks outnumbered the whites. In 1927 Marcus Garvey returned to Jamaica from the United States and he found a receptive audience for his Universal Negro Improvement Association (UNIA). The UNIA played a significant role in politicizing the masses, especially between 1928 and 1935, during Mary's early childhood years. Although formal political channels were closed to the majority of the black population, UNIA meetings served as training grounds for black working class activists and spokespersons. Garvey failed to win a seat in the legislature and left in 1935 for England. Despite numerous changes in the social and economic conditions of Jamaica, the political system in the 1930s continued to be closed to the majority of the island's population. In 1935, out of a population of 1,121,823, only 68,637 or a mere 6 percent were eligible to vote. Further political changes that ultimately led to self-government had their origins during the period of 1937–38 when poverty and unemployment were widespread. Work stoppages and disturbances increased throughout the island and came to a head in riots during May 1938. This crisis ultimately led to a different political order for Jamaica, largely as a result of the work of the Moyne Commission set up in 1938 to examine the causes of the riots. In 1944, a new constitution came into being, based on universal adult suffrage and limited self-government. Constitutional changes continued over the next decade, culminating in Jamaica's independence in 1962.[1]

From a social perspective Jamaica, like the other West Indian islands, was a stratified society. During the period of transition to independence, Jamaica was divided into three broad social classes: lower-class blacks, middle-class browns, and the upper-class whites. There were always blacks, browns and whites in each of the major classes but one colour was always predominant in each category. While there was no institutionalized colour line, the economic stratification by race was distinct. White domination in the civil service was so apparent that in 1943 only two of the island's highest twenty-five administrative officials were coloured Jamaicans. Most of these posts were held by English civil servants sent out for limited periods from Westminster. Race and colour were really shorthand designations of class. Similar relationships were found to exist between colour and such variables as income, literacy, education, family life, speech patterns and religion. In Kingston, the large stores, banks and commission houses were owned by whites; and the chief subordinate positions were held by browns.[2]

Neither ancestry nor appearance is wholly determinative in the West Indies, in that one can change one's 'colour' by acquiring education, manners, wealth and friends. Personal status and class affiliation can be altered through any of those factors. The rural peasantry and the urban proletariat were aware of the elite mores and were encouraged to emulate them. Education was, and still is, seen as the most potent mechanism for achieving status. The goal of schooling was to win prizes and to come out on top with an appropriate set of manners — speech, dress, deportment. If one was black and poor, one needed both prizes and manners to get far. Educational patterns reflected, validated and reinforced class differences.[3] Given this reality, it can be understood why Mary, who was born black, poor and living in a rural area, would be determined to acquire these assets to improve her prospects for the future. Her natural gift of brilliance was, of course, a central facilitating factor, coupled with an innate drive for achievement, a desire to move from the rural to the urban area where her potential could be reached, and a strong sense of nationalism.

Mary's Early Years

When Mary Jane Seivwright was born, there was no schooling beyond the primary level except for the wealthy. Jamaica's school system was deemed a pathetic exhibit of British failure. There was a universal fear, often privately expressed among dominant whites, that anything above the most elementary education would 'spoil' the black people. Primary education was an adjunct of the churches, mostly Anglican. In 1936 more than 50 percent of the children in Jamaica were not in regular attendance in primary school. Compulsory education laws were considered a farce because there were too few spaces for all to get into the schools, even if all decided to attend. Only about one-quarter of the population ever reached the fifth class in an elementary school, and only a handful ever reached the fee-charging secondary schools. Only 120,000 places were available in government schools for the 255,000 children between ages seven and fifteen.[4] Some of the children studied on their own with help from the teachers and then went to various centres to take the pupil teacher training examination. Like many clever country girls, Mary stayed on at the primary school and studied on her own and with the help of her teacher. Leleka Champagnie, a past president of the NAJ, came from the same village of Endeavour. Her sister attended primary school with Mary. Even at that early age, Mary's natural ability for high achievement was evident and she was considered to be "very bright". Leleka pointed out that her pastor was always telling her stories about Mary outshining him at school. Revd Luther Gibbs, a childhood classmate, recalled that

She was a very friendly person, very social, she was fond of all types of indoor games, like checkers, draughts, table-tennis, and then outdoor, she was not afraid of playing cricket and baseball, and of course, she was the star in all of that. She didn't want anybody to beat her and most times she came out on top. Mary was a bright student, diligent and hard working, no task was too difficult for her. In those days, most girls were afraid of mathematics, but Mary excelled at all of this. She was very good at mathematics.[5]

In primary school, Mary learned sewing and gardening, but her real love was gardening. She could not wait to get through the sewing to go to the garden. She had a small garden patch of peas, corn and other vegetables which her father gave to her and he helped her with the gardening. Her love of the land is central to the person she is today.

Mary's mother was a Baptist and her father an Anglican. The social divisions of Jamaican life were reflected in its religious-cultural divisions. Anglicanism was the faith of the established interests: the judiciary, education, medicine, political leadership and the economic elite. The masses espoused the folk culture and were generally transitional between African religions and formal Christianity.[6] Given the elitism that was attached to belonging to the established church, it was not surprising that Mary attended the Anglican church. It was one indicator of social status and would be a desirable choice for those aspiring to moving up the social scale. The minister, Revd J.S. Rowe, and Mary's teacher, Mr J.E. Brooks, soon recognized that Mary had much potential. As Mary puts it, "They said I was very brainy and to keep my brains active I continued studying and wrote the pupil teacher examinations three times." By the time that she was sixteen, Mary had completed writing those exams and she was the youngest pupil to take those exams. Her parents and the pastor wanted her to become a teacher. Revd Rowe was very helpful and eventually arranged for her to go to Brown's Town, also in St Ann but some distance away from where Mary lived, where he had relatives. Her parents supported her and she was allowed to live in the rectory where she did not have to pay rent. A caretaker 'adopted' her and helped her. At that young age of seventeen, Mary looked after herself, prepared her own meals and taught in the school.

To be poor, black and female severely limited her options in an era when there were few career choices open to women. Teaching was respectable and seen as a desirable option for a bright, young black woman. Schools were attached to the church and soon a vacancy occurred at Rio Bueno where the parish church was located and her pastor arranged for her to teach in the primary school there. Nursing, however, was always Mary's dream. She attributed this strong desire to an accident her father had one day while he was working on his farm. Mary explained: "He was a small farmer and we did not have a lot of level land and up in the Dry Harbour mountains, it is hilly and the farmers there do a lot of terracing so that the crops would not get washed away when the rains came. They were good wall builders – the farmers in my section of St Ann – those nice stone walls around pastures . . . And while he was building the wall a stone rolled down and fell on his foot. Now he had on heavy farmers boots but the stone rolled down and picked up speed with a force enough to crush his small toe in the shoe. He had to go to hospital to have the toe amputated."

He was sent to St Dacre's Hospital in St Ann, some distance away from their village. Her mother sent Mary, just ten years old, with a cousin to visit her father. When Mary arrived, the doctor came to attend to her father and the curtains were drawn around his bed. Mary reminisced: "When I got there my father was trembling and I saw him with tears in his eyes and I said 'Pappy, what is happening?' And he said, 'The doctor tear the dressing off. But when the nurses come, they use a basin and cotton and squeeze lotion and then with tweezers, they lift the dressing off and it is so much easier. God bless the nurses.' " That incident and those remarks planted the seed for nursing in young Mary's mind. One particular nurse and her kind treatment of her father further added to this enchantment. Mary described how impressed she was with this nurse's uniform. "And when I looked at her she had on this beautiful fall. She had a blue uniform with a white apron and this white fall and she made such an impression. To me the fall and the way it fitted, it made her look like an angel. And my father had used those words that the nurse was an angel of mercy. And from that I began to feel good about the nurse."

From that time, Mary began to notice people who were suffering and had sympathy for them. She and each of her sisters had animals of their own which they tended – chickens and a goat each. Whenever any mishap occurred to any of the animals, Mary would take care of it and "began to play nurse at everything".

The final incident that confirmed for Mary her decision to enter nursing was, "One day when a beautiful lady came to the school and she was dressed in a brownish uniform . . . I found out that she was a public health nurse who had come to teach health care to the children. Then and there I made up my mind, yes I was going to be a nurse and nothing would stop me. But I did not want to be a hospital nurse, I wanted to be like this lady so that I could teach as well as taking care of people."

Her determination was evident from an early age when she was studying on her own for the pupil teacher examinations. She was adamant that she would wait for "the moment when I could get away from my parents to switch to nursing". In those days, students could not enter nursing before the age of twenty-one. Mary patiently waited and continued teaching at Rio Bueno Elementary School until she applied to enter nursing. She was sent to the distant town of Falmouth for her physical examination and was deemed to be in good health. During the physical examination, the doctor had asked her a number of anatomy questions to which Mary responded correctly. The nursing programme was due to start in January and Mary would be twenty-one in the following April. The physician wrote a letter of recommendation to the nursing school indicating that although Mary was not twenty-one, she was quite mature and bright and that he would recommend that she be admitted. This impressed Miss Alice Walton, the matron of Kingston Public Hospital, and consequently Mary was admitted to the programme a few months before attaining the prescribed age.

Her Start in Nursing

At the turn of the century, nurses were relegated to a lower stratum by virtue of the stigma attached to the service they performed, their gender and the fact that they were black or coloured colonials. The long hours of arduous work, poor accommodation, minimal remuneration for services, limited recreation time and rigid discipline meant that recruitment and retention of nurses remained a grave concern for the authorities. Middle and upper class members of the society avoided hospitals and hired private nurses. Nurses who received training at the public hospital in Kingston quickly found employment in the homes of the wealthy, leaving the hospitals poorly staffed.

At the end of the 1920s, public health remained unsatisfactory, with the incidence of diseases such as malaria, hookworm, tuberculosis, yaws and venereal diseases high. Other diseases included dysentery, typhoid fever, pneumonia and yellow fever. Despite the variety of communicable diseases that were prevalent among the poor and coloured population, knowledge of such diseases, of public health and of nutrition were lacking and noticeably absent from the curriculum. Such omission from the curriculum reflected the class and racial biases of the colonialists where the curriculum was irrelevant to the needs of most of the local people. There were three established training schools for nurses in Kingston: the Kingston Public Hospital that provided a three-year programme for general trained nurses; the Nuttall Nursing Home, a private institution that trained general nurses; and the Victoria Jubilee Lying-In Hospital that trained midwives for nine months. Student nurses who received training in rural hospitals were required to receive additional training at the Kingston Public Hospital prior to examinations in order to attain higher standards for certification.[7]

By 1944, when Mary was ready to enter nursing, decentralization of training was being introduced. Mary entered St James General Hospital (now Cornwall Regional Hospital) in Montego Bay with a batch of twelve student nurses. She spent the first year there and finished at the top of her class. Enid Fuller, a graduate nurse at that hospital when Mary was a student nurse there, spoke highly of her excellent care. She was particularly impressed that Mary, with all her accomplishments, was "the same person" who did not forget her early roots or her religion. The second and third years of Mary's training were spent at the Kingston Public Hospital. The English matron at that time was Miss Alice Walton. She initiated several educational reforms for the training of nurses during her tenure at the public hospital. Many stories circulated among the probationers about Miss Walton's tough reputation. Mary tells the tale that "some of us were scared, others of us were brave and ready to take her on. I was one of those who thought that I had begun to love this profession and I am not going to allow any matron to turn me off." A telling example of Mary's dogged determination that no one would stand in her way of achieving her goal.

During Mary's apprenticeship, lectures were given by physicians and at their convenience. Trainees were expected to attend lectures despite a twelve-hour night shift, and even if they were scheduled to work in the afternoon. When students were scheduled for lectures, they were expected to complete their assignments before leaving for the lectures, so as to ensure minimum disruption for those left behind to assume the additional assignments. Despite these hardships, Mary said, "I look back on those years with a lot of joy. It was very pleasant and I began to love nursing." The matrons were all British and were responsible for the training of the student nurses. It was an apprenticeship system; the hospital relied on its trainees to provide service. The patriarchal race and class system prevailed, with the male physicians holding power both in terms of the training of student nurses and in the administration of the hospital. Next were the white female British matrons and, at the bottom, were the black and brown female Jamaican staff nurses and the student nurses. Some opportunities for advancement to middle management positions as ward sisters or as matrons of the small rural hospitals were afforded the local Jamaican nurses. However, they were never given permanent appointments as matrons of the three large hospitals in Kingston.

In the early 1940s nursing was still largely unorganized and lacking leadership or a voice in its own affairs. However, prior to Mary's entry into nursing, several events had taken place which were to have positive results for nursing and consequently for Mary.

The riots of the 1930s and the formation of organized labour among the working class had its impact on nursing. While nurses did not join the trade unions, they began formulating plans for a professional organization. The 1938 Moyne Commission had issued its report and health reform was a major concern among its recommendations. The upgrading of health programmes was seen as a top priority. By 1943 the secretary of state for the colonies had appointed the Rushcliffe Commission to examine training for nurses who were to serve in colonial territories. The commission was also requested to make recommendations having regard for the need in those territories for increased public health activities and for the fostering and development of community welfare. Two subcommittees were formed: one was to examine "the training of nurses in the United Kingdom and the Dominions for service in colonial territories", the other was to examine "the training given in the colonies to indigenous nurses".

The outcome was a further recommendation to appoint two nurses to investigate conditions of training for nurses in the West Indies. With World War II in progress, there were delays and not until 1946 were Emily MacManus and Blanche Shenton sent by the Colonial Office to look into nursing conditions in the colonies. They readily recognized the lack of an educational programme and of qualified staff to implement one. They reported that "some Matrons and Hospital Authorities have made efforts to improvise, but most hospitals are already short of general accommodation and have been reluctant to acknowledge the fact that a successful nursing school must have rooms set apart for teaching and study purposes".[8] They strongly urged that hospital programmes establish preliminary training schools for student nurses and that candidates entering should have secondary school education with school certificates or should be able to pass a pre-admission examination. Recommendations were also made regarding accommodation for students and the need for sister tutors. These recommendations were not new, however, as the local leaders had already expressed similar views.

Also in 1946 Mary, then in the second year of her training, was fortunate enough to be present at the formation of the JGTNA, a milestone in nursing history in the island. Nita Barrow became the first president. Mary shared the excitement and significance of the occasion and recognized, as all the rank-and-file nurses did, that here was an opportunity for local leaders to emerge and promote the interests of Jamaican nurses. In 1947 Mary completed her nursing programme training. She would not benefit from any of the proposed educational changes, but she was adjudged the most outstanding student in her graduating class. Miss Walton had proposed that the girls who came first, second and third that year would be entitled to do midwifery, if they so desired. At that time nurses usually practised for a number of years before applying to do midwifery. Even so, they had no guarantee of being accepted as there was often a long waiting list. However, Mary, having topped her class and with the influence of the matron, immediately went on to the Victoria Jubilee Hospital for the nine-month midwifery training. Again she emerged at the top of her class, then chose to work for one year at the maternity hospital and develop her midwifery skills.

Public Health Nurse

Mary had never forgotten the public health nurse who had visited her school, nor had she lost her desire to work in the community. She had seen pregnant mothers dying from malnutrition in her village as she grew up and babies dying for want of care. She wanted to return to the village to teach her people, just like the nurse who had inspired her to make nursing her career. She entered the West Indies School of Public Health from which she graduated in 1949, again at the top of her class. Mary's triple first – in nursing, midwifery and public health nursing – is said to be unequalled to this day. It is interesting to note that Nita Barrow had been appointed to the School of Public Health not long before and she was Mary's tutor. The two were very different but they would become central and critical figures in the history of nursing in Jamaica and in the West Indian colonies in general. Even in their appearance they presented contrasting images. Nita Barrow was short and plump, little above five feet in height, while Mary was a tall, well-built, imposing woman, about six feet tall.

When Mary graduated from the School of Public Health, there was a dire need for qualified nurses with public health training not only in Jamaica but throughout the West Indies, as can be seen in the many official reports into health conditions in the colonies.[9] The School of Public Health and the nursing schools were looking for the best and brightest nurses from the West Indies to provide them with advanced training at the public health school. Lola Bragg, who was working at the Victoria Jubilee Hospital at the same time that Mary went there to do her midwifery, said that both of them had been selected for public health training and that Mary "was quite a brilliant lady, young woman. She was like a teacher herself in that class." Their friendship blossomed and has continued to the present day.

After completing public health training, the nurses were posted to various parishes across the island. Mary was assigned to Morant Bay, St Thomas. Her prize for being the top of the class was a government loan to purchase a car. In recounting this, Mary sounded quite thrilled and proud. She never forgot her first car, a brown and beige Hillman Minx. Even to own a car in the 1940s was an unusual occurrence and even more so when the owner was a young black junior nurse. She worked in St Thomas for five years as a public health nurse, responsible for pre- and postnatal supervision, maternal and child health supervision, school hygiene, communicable disease control programmes, and supervision of district midwives in home delivery service. During Mary's first year in St Thomas, the registration bill that the nurses had been promoting and working assiduously on since 1946 was finally passed in August 1951. Mary would certainly have been aware of the implications of this bill for the standards of nursing in Jamaica.

When she had almost completed five years of service in St Thomas, Mary began to look ahead. A nurses' exchange programme had been introduced for registered nurses to continue further studies abroad. Her thirst for further knowledge impelled her to grasp such an opportunity. She applied and in 1954 became the first Jamaican nurse to take advantage of the programme. She chose to go to New York and registered at Teachers' College, Columbia University, where she pursued a Bachelor of Science degree. Since the University Hospital had recently opened at Mona, there was the distinct possibility of a school of nursing being opened there. Astute as Mary was, she must have envisioned being considered to head the hospital and thus the programme.

In her first year, Mary worked for the first year as a public health nurse for the Visiting Nurse Services of New York. Her extensive community experience in the islands equipped her well to take on this new job in a different country. In fact, the responsibilities were fewer but, while less demanding, they were quite challenging. She was able to utilize her rich experience in maternal and child health supervision, and she was able to practise her skills in bedside nursing care, physical therapy and rehabilitation. In her second year, Mary moved to the Francis Delafield Hospital as a staff nurse and team leader on the cancer unit. This experience further strengthened her clinical skills as well as her leadership abilities. In that role, Mary gave direct nursing care to patients, medical and surgical, in various stages of illness, supervised the auxiliary personnel giving care, and conducted team conferences regarding the care of patients. During the course of her studies, Mary was appointed President's Scholar and received a full scholarship for tuition in her final semester. In 1956 she graduated with a Bachelor of Science with a major in nursing education.

Armed with her degree, further knowledge and the experience of living abroad, Mary returned to her native land only to be posted as a public health nurse to the remote village of Junction in the parish of St Elizabeth. This posting must have come as quite a shock and disappointment to Mary. She had returned with a degree and wider nursing experience only to be given no credit for her achievements. There are differing opinions as to why she was posted to that remote community, having returned more qualified than most nurses at that time. It has been suggested that the British postgraduate training was still held in high esteem although the United States and Canada were at that time in the forefront of providing higher education at university level for nurses. North America was moving ahead with innovative changes for nursing education – witness Nita Barrow's experience in Canada. Unfortunately, those in authority in Jamaica at that time were strongly British in attitude and prone to dismiss the North American system as 'inferior'. Another view is that senior nurses were not too pleased with Mary's experience and there was jealousy about her degree, a rarity for nurses at the time. Indeed, it is doubtful whether any other Jamaican or West Indian nurse had a bachelor's degree in 1956. She most certainly was unique. It has been said that many of the senior personnel often talked about her – that she was ambitious and wanted to advance in professional nursing. As one of her colleagues pointed out, "They made it difficult for her." This is not too unusual or unexpected as, traditionally in nursing, the younger, more educated nurses generally are 'given a rough time' by their seniors with fewer academic qualifications than they have. They are seen as a threat to their seniors. In Canada and the United States, the introduction of baccalaureate-prepared nurses in health care institutions encountered much hostility from those who were diploma-prepared. As late as the 1990s in Canada, this tension between university-prepared and college-prepared nurses has continued. The latter claim that they have more 'hands-on' experience and greater practical skills than the university graduates and often criticize them. "We eat our young" is a commonly heard expression in nursing.

While she was working at Junction, Mary found a haven at the home of Lola Bragg in Kingston. She would work in the rural area during the week and visit Lola's family at weekends and other times. The Bragg family were Mary's strong supporters, especially Dr Percy Bragg, who was a dentist. He encouraged Mary in everything that she did and had boosted her morale when she was working in Junction. He would say to her, "Go for it, Mary. Go for it!"

Mary was obviously not happy with her posting to the rural area where she felt, and rightly so, that her newly acquired knowledge and skills were not properly utilized. Given the state of the art in nursing education in Jamaica in the 1950s, where there was a desperate need for well-qualified nurses as tutors, the issue of appropriate use of qualified personnel could be raised. Clearly gender was not an issue here and so was it race? By the 1950s, the colonial administrators were aware that they needed to promote local nurses to senior positions, especially since the UCHWI was already operational. It would seem logical that Mary, having returned to Jamaica from the United States armed with a degree in nursing education as her major, would be a prime candidate for a position at the School of Public Health. But it was not to be. The West Indian nurses who had gone to Great Britain for advanced training during the war years returned and were assigned to UCHWI or the School of Public Health.

By this time, there were quite a few black nurses in leadership positions; the professional association had been received into full membership of the ICN since 1953, and there was a concerted effort by nurses in the West Indies to get together to share their strengths and overcome their weaknesses. Nita Barrow was at that time the matron of the UCHWI and its School of Nursing and was subsequently appointed the principal nursing officer in Jamaica. Race, then, did not appear to be the central issue. What was it then?

One of Mary's junior colleagues recollected that she had first heard about Mary in connection with public health nursing. She had been the focus of discussion among the public health nurses because she had reputedly parked her car at the airport when she left for New York. The Ministry of Health gave all public health nurses a loan to purchase cars for use in the performance of their duties, as most of these communities were in the rural areas and transportation was a major problem. The cars belonged ultimately to the ministry until the loans were repaid. On her departure for Columbia University, Mary, fiercely independent, used her famous, or now infamous, Hillman Minx to get to the airport and left the car there unattended for the ministry's office to pick up. This behaviour was considered to be defiant, to say the least, and invited controversy. Whenever her name came up in the course of conversation with nurses, her action became a mantra: "You're speaking about Mary Jane who left the car at the airport!" It is believed by many that the Ministry of Health had punished her for that action by banishing her to Junction, a junior assignment, when there were more senior positions – principal nursing officer, for example – available at that time. Mary certainly was not happy with her posting and indeed, it was an inappropriate use of her wealth of knowledge and experience. The power of the Ministry of Health in determining Mary's fate was clearly evident. She had to be taught a lesson – to toe the line and to be punished. Lola Bragg observed in her gentle manner, 'It was fate [because] they could have found other places for her with her degree and all that . . . but I don't think that all nursing was happy."[10] This did not imply that being sent to a rural area was a form of punishment, but Mary already had five years of community experience before going abroad and, furthermore, she was replacing a junior nurse who was leaving to do her public health training! Clearly it was a misuse of her talents and, in that sense, could be construed as punishment. It was also a poor deployment of qualified staff, and a failure to recognize and reward excellence. The colonial attitude still persisted!

Lucy Flash O'Sullivan, the junior nurse in Junction who was replaced by Mary, told me about their first meeting. Mary did not seem to be enthusiastic about meeting the senior staff of the parish in the town of Black River, not far away, even though she knew them. Lucy had asked her, " 'So what do you plan? . . . How do you propose to deal with this seclusion and with your wealth of experience and exposure? What do you see as the very necessary changes in an area like this?' Having listened to what I said about the area, she said, well, she thinks that the best way to spend her time is to reorganize the office her way. She thinks that is the best that she can do. And that she would take it from there. I found it very interesting because I realized that would not last very long, and that she would not be sticking to that job too long. I was trying to find out from her why she would agree to take this position, which in my estimation was probably the lowest position in the system for someone with her qualifications."[11]

And, indeed, Mary would not stay long in that post. It was not what she had wanted nor what she had expected. Dissatisfied, Mary remained there for one year until August 1957. It was not a happy time for her. Her abilities were not being utilized or acknowledged. She felt restless and it seemed that she was searching, trying to find the right place, the right job, the right thing to do. Eventually, she decided that she wanted to see what life was like in Canada. For a year she worked as a public health nurse with the City Department of Health in Toronto, but she found the climate much too cold. Once more, she set off for New York, this time to pursue a Master of Arts degree with a major in nursing education at Teachers' College, her alma mater.

Mary's area of specialization was supervision and administration in public health nursing services. She returned to Francis Delafield Hospital for her internship as a nursing service supervisor in cancer nursing. This clinical practice exposed her to an intensive and invaluable experience. She supervised and evaluated the nursing care given by all categories of health workers – registered nurses, practical nurses and auxiliary personnel – and supervised the head nurses in ward management. Six weeks in the office of the director of nursing followed, in order to gain a perspective of organizational management. Finally, she had to teach for six weeks in an in-service education programme for auxiliary personnel. Once again, Mary was selected as President's Scholar and received a fully paid tuition scholarship toward the completion of her master's degree. On completion of this well-rounded practical and theoretical curriculum at Teachers' College, Mary graduated with a Master of Arts degree in January 1960.

After completing her studies, Mary dreamed of returning to Jamaica to serve in a position where she could make the greatest contribution to her country. She had maintained her links and her nursing connections with longstanding friends while she was abroad, in particular with Lola Bragg and Leleka Champagnie. They were excellent contacts as they too were to hold positions of power in nursing and each would serve as presidents of the NAJ. Through her friends, Mary kept up to date with events in Jamaica and in the West Indies as a whole. She was determined to return when a position became available that she felt would utilize her abilities and give her the opportunity to make an impact on nursing education and so help her people and her country. The time was not yet ready, but the groundwork was being laid.

Nursing Research Project Director

In July 1961 Mary was offered the position of nursing research project director at the Institute of Research and Service in Nursing Education at Teachers' College. This international project consisted of a series of international cross-cultural studies in nursing and was sponsored by the college and financed by the US Public Health Service. The chief investigator was Dr Leo W. Simmons. Mary's role would be to introduce, explain and gain approval for the project in Jamaica, which had been chosen as one of the sites for the project. She would also select and train interviewers and direct the data collection. This offer seemed ideal for Mary since she would be able to return to Jamaica as a researcher in nursing. The purpose of the project was to examine the vocational images and coping patterns of public health nurses and it was the first of its kind to be conducted in Jamaica.

The possibility that Mary might be offered the post brought her and Nita Barrow together again. Nita was the principal nursing officer in Jamaica at the time, and her permission and cooperation were among those required before the project could come into effect. Apparently, there were some reservations about offering the post to Mary. Correspondence between 1960 and 1961 between Dr Simmons and Nita Barrow suggests that there was some concern about Mary's suitability for the project. This seemed to be related to her interpersonal style rather than to her academic or research qualifications. In a letter from Teachers' College, dated 4 February 1961, Dr Simmons reported on a meeting he had in Kingston with Mary and Nita:

A very frank and forthright discussion was held between Miss Barrow, Miss Seivwright and myself, in which we reviewed our past relationships and endeavoured to clear up certain misunderstandings, to point out some of the errors in judgment or action that we have made either separately or together, and to reach a better basis of communication for our future work together. This session was extremely helpful to me . . . During the pilot phase of the project, July and August, of this year, I shall accept responsibility for reaching a decision on the capacity and qualifications of Miss Seivwright to serve as Project director for the major portion of the programme. I feel I should state now, however, that, so far, I have found no one, either in Jamaica or at the University here where Miss Seivwright has been a student for several years who really questions her intellectual ability and training capacity for an assignment like this one, especially with some careful guidance, and if or when she can be fitted into the programme comfortably and effectively, I shall lend every effort to make this possible . . . Personally, I also want to commend Miss Nita Barrow for the part she played during the past week in helping to achieve what was for me a happy outcome of my second visit to Jamaica.[12]

Dr Simmons did reach his decision in July. The position of nursing research project director was offered to Mary and she accepted it.

The NAJ provided an office for the project at their headquarters in Trevennion Road, and from there Mary conducted the research, distributed questionnaires and collated the information. While she was in Jamaica, she stayed at Lola Bragg's family home in Kingston. Whenever Dr Simmons or senior staff with the project visited Jamaica, the Braggs entertained them and even hosted a cocktail party for them. As Lola said, "[It was] because we were family. So as a family we felt like we were a family to her. That's the closeness we had as friends. You know we just had to do this right."

While Mary was working with the nursing project in Kingston, the possibility of developing a university programme for registered nurses was at an embryonic stage. Mary used her research skills to gather information from the Ministry of Health that could identify nursing needs in terms of service and education because she knew that most nurses who would attend such a university programme would come from the government sector. At the same time, she renewed her contact with Leleka Champagnie who had also been abroad, pursuing her nursing studies in England. She mentioned to Leleka that she wanted to return home and asked her to keep her informed about any future job opportunities.

Mary worked with the research project in Jamaica until December 1962 when it was completed. The following year, she remained with the Institute of Research and Service in New York as a research assistant, coding, tabulating, and analysing the data, and writing the research report. This experience enhanced Mary's research skills and nurtured her love for research. It was inevitable that Mary would eventually turn to further postgraduate education. By 1964 she enrolled in the Doctor of Education programme at Teachers' College in New York, with nursing education as her major, and curriculum and teaching in collegiate nursing education (public health) as her special area. She had already been inducted into two honour societies of Teachers' College in 1963. These societies are status organizations and two memberships would have been very important to Mary. They were indicators that would assign her to a particular social class, something that colour alone could, and did, preclude in the colour/class conditions existing then in Jamaican society. She was steadily moving up the social ladder.

Chief Project Nurse

In order to survive, during the first three years of her doctoral studies, Mary worked part-time as a nursing supervisor at the Hebrew Hospital for the Chronic Sick in the Bronx, primarily a geriatric institution. She supervised registered nurses, practical nurses and auxiliary workers in the provision of care for the elderly and chronically ill patients. However, her academic work did not suffer. She received a third scholarship, having been selected as Dean's Scholar and was awarded fully paid tuition for the spring semester of 1966. After completing all coursework in the spring of 1967, Mary took up a new appointment as chief project nurse with the Comprehensive Child Care Project at the Albert Einstein College of Medicine at the Montefiore Hospital and Medical Centre in the Bronx from 1967 to 1969.

The nature of the project was all-encompassing, as its title suggests. It entailed the development of protocols and job descriptions for nursing and auxiliary personnel, as well as directing and supervising project nurses. Curriculum development and training programmes for new categories of health workers and in-service programmes for current workers were other aspects of the position. Mary welcomed the opportunity to become involved with the development of policies and procedures for interagency cooperation and coordination, and to serve as a member of the interdisciplinary central staff of the project. It also allowed her to organize and direct community health education programmes. For eight months of her time with the childcare project, Mary acted as a nursing education consultant to the Adelphi University School of Nursing in Long Island. Here she worked with faculty in developing and implementing a four-credit course in community nursing within a Master of Arts degree programme. The size and scope of these activities would overwhelm most, but not Mary. She pushed herself to the limit in an endless pursuit of excellence, exemplifying the concept that J.W. Gardner argued for so eloquently: "We must foster a conception of excellence that may be applied to every degree of ability and to every socially acceptable activity . . . We need excellent physicists and excellent mechanics . . . The tone and fibre of our society depend upon a pervasive and almost universal striving for good performance."[13] Excellence was Mary's endless mission for herself and for others no less. The mastery of research, teaching and administrative skills were to serve Mary well when the time came for her to use them in Jamaica. That time was slow in arriving, but arrive it did.

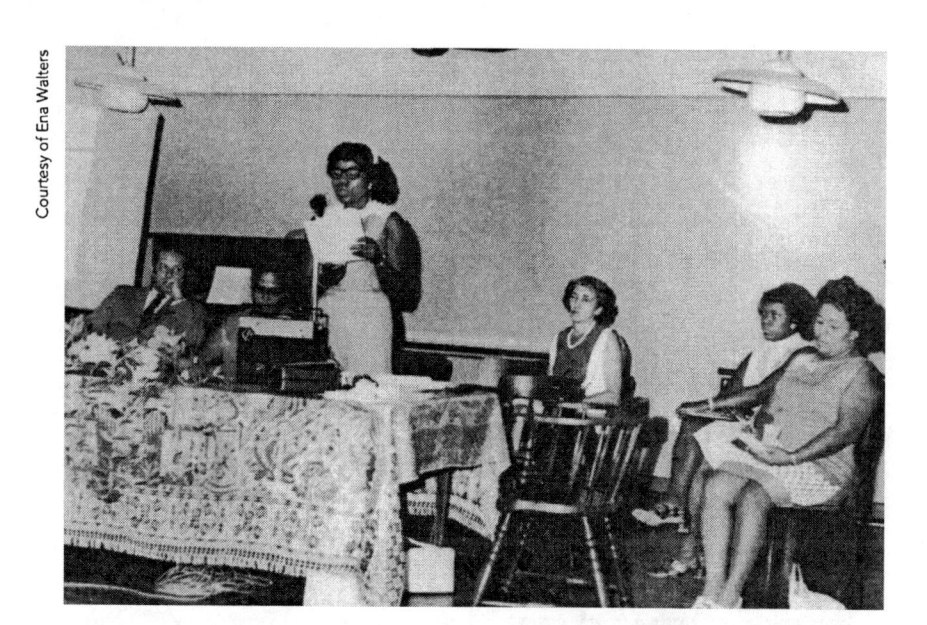

Summer school, Kingston, Jamaica, 1969. From left to right, Dr H. Eldmire, minister of health; Lola Bragg, president of the Nurses' Association of Jamaica; Mary (standing); Gertrude Swaby; Gladys Lewis; Carmen Brooks

In the meantime, several significant events occurred in the West Indies while Mary was away. The newly formed Federation of the West Indies between 1958 and 1961 greatly facilitated regional cooperation of both a governmental and nongovernmental nature in nursing. The nongovernmental CNO was inaugurated at a conference in Antigua in 1957; the first nursing administrators' conference (governmental) was held in 1959 in Barbados; a survey of the twenty-three schools of nursing was initiated in 1965; and a regional nursing body was being advocated in 1970. Mary maintained a visible and vital presence in these developments. She attended the meetings of the CNO held biennially in different islands and was invited by the executive of the NAJ (her friend Leleka Champagnie was then the president) to deliver the opening address of the nineteenth annual summer school of the NAJ held in August 1967 at Mary Seacole House, the then headquarters of both the NAJ and the Nursing Council. The content of Mary's speech gave a view of some of the fundamental beliefs of this woman: self-actualization, professional accountability, and community service. In her words: "You will strive vigorously toward what you are capable of becoming." It was her conviction that "if you are committed to your profession, it is expected that you will make it your life-work; you will be proud to belong; do all in your power to enhance its status, and do nothing to bring it in disrepute". Finally, she advocated identification and involvement with the wider community: "You must feel that you have a personal stake in its future, because you are an important part of it . . . Isolation should be replaced with active and meaningful participation in community affairs."[14]

INTERNATIONAL NURSING ADVISOR

In 1969 Mary Seivwright marked up a first again. She was the first West Indian nurse to be employed as a nurse advisor at ICN headquarters in Geneva, Switzerland. The nursing world has a good communication network regarding leadership potential candidates. Mary had become well known both in the United States and the Caribbean, having written as well as given addresses. Her experience as director of the Nursing Research Project was also an asset. Moreover, she was well-prepared clinically as well as educationally and one of the few with such advanced qualifications from the Caribbean. It proved to be an excellent choice.

When she was appointed advisor to the ICN, the *Daily Gleaner,* the leading Jamaican newspaper, surveyed her accomplishments and appointment in its issue of 20 March 1969.

Mary worked with the ICN from 1969 to 1971. In 1969, following the fourteenth quadrennial congress of the ICN in Montreal, the Jamaican delegation hosted a reception in her honour to celebrate her most recent achievement – a doctoral degree. Theresa Boyne, the registrar of the Nursing Council of Jamaica in 1996, recollected her first encounter with Mary on that joyous occasion. Speaking to her colleagues, Mary had shared with them her motivation to achieve her doctoral degree. She had been driven by her philosophy that "Whatever a man can do, she's convinced that a woman can do it and perhaps better. And whatever a white woman can do, a black woman can do it. And whatever any woman can do, a nurse can do it and perhaps do it better. I'll never forget that. And I think that she lived out her philosophy."

In her role as ICN advisor, Mary used her administrative skills to assist national nursing associations in member countries in various ways, depending on their needs. Among these were the formulation of nursing legislation; social and economic welfare of their members; nursing education or research consultation

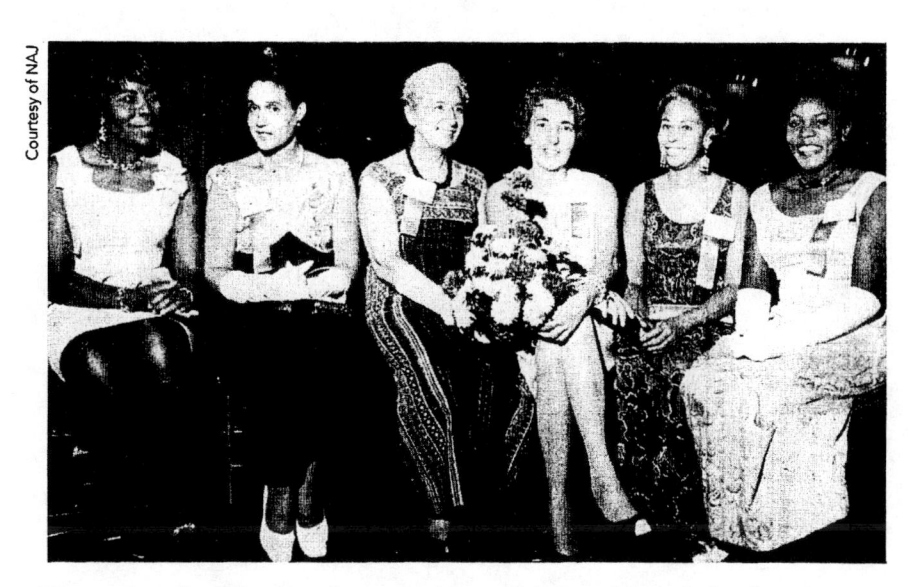

Fourteenth quadrennial congress, International Council of Nurses, Montreal, Canada, 1969

services. She represented the ICN at international meetings and acted as recording secretary at ICN standing or special committees. She also prepared professional papers for the organization when required. To be an advisor with the ICN was a much envied position and exposed her to a wide range of international contacts.

Her consultations brought her to the Caribbean, where she represented the ICN at the Commonwealth Caribbean Nurses Meeting in Barbados in April 1970, and was a member of a committee set up to prepare a budget for the administrative expenses for that meeting, and the travel costs for the participants. That meeting was historic as the Commonwealth Foundation provided a grant to enable the nurses of the region to carry out further studies on the methodology of establishing a regional nursing body. Such a body had been advocated since 1959 when the notion of a Federation of the West Indies was proposed. The Regional Nursing Body was finally formed and it has played and continues to play a critical part in Caribbean nursing. It meets annually in a different West Indian territory.

In May 1970 she visited the Nurses' Association of Dominica. During her brief visit, she paid a courtesy call on the governor, His Excellency Sir Louis Cools-Lartigue, and met with other government officials, including the minister of education and health and the chief medical officer. She spent the two days working with the Professional Nursing Association, met their executive body and held a general

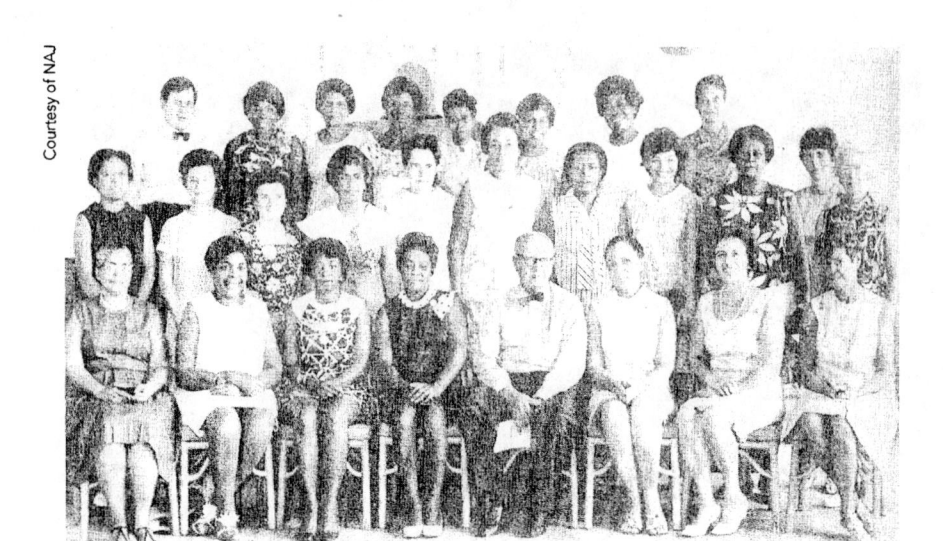

Delegates to the Commonwealth nursing seminar, 1970. Front row, seated, Nita Barrow (second from left) and Helen Mussallem (second from right). Standing, second row, is Mary Jane Seivwright (second from left)

meeting for the nurses in the island. She was also invited by her Jamaican nursing colleagues to deliver the opening address for the first island conference of the NAJ.

Mary's colleagues knew that it was always her desire to return to Jamaica. It was Leleka who informed Mary that the position of director of the Advanced Nursing Unit at UWI was to be filled and suggested that if she were interested she should apply. The position was advertised in the *Daily Gleaner* of 6 December 1970 and Mary applied from Geneva on 15 December 1970. A formal letter of appointment as director in advanced nursing education, Department of Social and Preventive Medicine, was offered to her in a letter dated 5 March 1971, signed by the registrar of the university. Dr Kenneth Standard, professor and head of the Department of Social and Preventive Medicine, also wrote to Mary welcoming her and assuring her that as director of the Nursing Unit, she would have full control of the programme and his support whenever needed.

When Mary took up her new appointment in April 1971, she entered a new phase in her life. She was first once more: the first nurse in the West Indies to hold a doctoral degree and the first West Indian nurse to head a West Indian university nursing programme. This was no mean accomplishment. Finally, her dream of being in a leadership position in her own country and among her own people where she could effect change for the betterment of her community had been realized.

NOTES

1. Abigail B. Bakan, *Ideology and Class Conflict in Jamaica* (Montreal: McGill-Queen's University Press, 1990), 68–98; see also George Hunte, *Jamaica* (London: B.T. Batsford, 1976), 81–113, for an account of emancipation to modern times.
2. P. Blanshard, *Democracy and Empire in the Caribbean* (New York: Macmillan), 86–87; D. Lowenthal, *West Indian Societies* (London: Oxford University Press, 1972), 81–117.
3. Lowenthal, *West Indian Societies*, 134–38.
4. Blanshard, *Democracy and Empire*, 101.
5. *Profiles: Mary Jane Seivwright* (Jamaica Information Service, videotape, 1990).
6. G. Lewis, *The Growth of the Modern West Indies* (New York: Monthly Review Press, 1968), 194–95.
7. P. Hay Ho Sang, "The Development of Nursing Education in Jamaica, West Indies: 1900–1975" (DEd diss., Teachers' College, Columbia University, 1984), 92–94.
8. *Report of the Committee on the Training of Nurses for the Colonies*, Cmd. 6672 (1945), 3, 8, cited in Ho Sang, "The Development of Nursing Education", 176.
9. *Colonial Officer, West India Royal Commission Report*, Cmd. 6607 (June 1945); *Report of the Committee on the Training of Nurses*.
10. Lola Bragg, personal interview, June 1996. All material quoted from Lola Bragg is from this interview.
11. Lucy Flash O'Sullivan, personal interview, June 1996. All material quoted from O'Sullivan is from this interview.
12. Letter from Dr Leo Simmons to Nita Barrow, 8 February 1961 (History of Nursing Archives, series 6, Institute of Research and Service in Nursing Education, subseries 4, Research and Consultation Grants, Columbia University, Teachers' College, Department of Nursing, 1983, Microfiche #3398).
13. J.W. Gardner, *Excellence: Can We Be Equal and Excellent Too?* (New York: Harper and Row, 1962), 131–32.
14. M.J. Seivwright, "You, Your Profession and the Community", *Jamaican Nurse* 7 (1967): 6–7, 31.

CHAPTER SIX

An Extraordinary Woman

The appointment of Dr Mary Jane Seivwright as director of the Advanced Nursing Education Unit (ANEU) in the Faculty of Medical Sciences at UWI was a major accomplishment for her, for the nation, and for the Caribbean as a whole. A Caribbean nurse had finally achieved the prestigious leadership position of a university nursing programme. One of Mary's many students, Marina Andrewin Staine, who is now a clinical nurse specialist and coordinator of a corrections health care centre in Florida, described the excitement among the young neophyte nurses when Mary returned to head the ANEU at UWI. "The rumour was around about this Jamaican lady who had a PhD. At that time, nurses with degrees, much less nurses with PhDs, was [sic] an almost unknown . . . I was intrigued and I went to a talk that she had just to have a look at her . . . For us as students, new graduates, this was somebody extraordinary. We never met anybody with a PhD. A few people had BScNs but masters' [degrees] were very rare. So a PhD was an extraordinary person . . . She was the first nurse that I ever met with a doctorate."[1] Thelma Campbell, coordinator of the Nurse Practitioner Programme, smiled as she recalled, "We were all so proud of her when she arrived from the States. We all rushed to every meeting to hear her as the first Jamaican and the first West Indian [nurse] with a PhD. I felt that we were at the feet of the master!"[2]

The Advanced Nursing Education Unit

Before the Advanced Nursing Education Programme was introduced at UWI, Caribbean nurses who wished to obtain post-basic preparation in teaching and administration had to travel to Great Britain or North America. Some of them never returned; some of those who did return had obvious difficulty readjusting to the local situation. Post-basic education within the Caribbean setting was seen as the best solution to the problem. After several years of discussion, starting with the first meeting of regional nursing leaders in 1959, the ANEU was established in October 1966 with the implementation of a programme leading to a Certificate in Nursing Administration and a Certificate in Nursing Education. The programmes were conducted in accordance with an agreement signed in 1965 by the Jamaican government, UWI and PAHO. The programme would offer post-basic education and training, relevant to the region, to senior Caribbean nurses in the functional areas of nursing administration and education so as to enable them to function as mid-level administrators and managers of nursing services, and as tutors in the schools of nursing.

The ANEU was attached to the Department of Social and Preventive Medicine, which seemed a logical choice as it was the only department that had nurses working in it involved in a community health programme with a nearby community. From the very outset, the two post-basic courses offered by the unit were seen as the first step in a long-range plan for the development of higher education for nurses of the region and for the improvement of health care in the Caribbean. It commenced operation on 3 October 1966 with a PAHO/WHO consultant, Dr Rae Chittick, a Canadian nurse, as director.

A two-year pilot project was launched in 1966, financed by PAHO/WHO and the governments of Bahamas, Barbados, Grenada, Jamaica, and Trinidad and Tobago, with PAHO providing technical assistance as well. The programme began with sixteen students from six territories: Antigua, Barbados, Grenada, Guyana, Jamaica, and Trinidad and Tobago. Nine of these candidates enrolled in the nursing education certificate course, with seven choosing the nursing administration option.

The ANEU, funded at that time on an annual basis, soon began to make an impact. The participants at the Nursing Education Seminar held in April 1968 in Guyana recommended that a degree programme be developed at UWI. This need was also recognized by the Caribbean health ministers at their first meeting in February 1969 in Port of Spain, Trinidad.

In its third year of operation, a comprehensive evaluation of the certificate programme was conducted by a PAHO/WHO consultant, Dr Marlene Kramer from the University of California, San Francisco. She also advised and assisted the ANEU faculty on the development of an initial draft proposal for a post-basic bachelor's degree in nursing as the second step in the educational development plan.

At the end of the first five years of the existence of the ANEU, more than one hundred senior Caribbean nurses in the two certificate programmes had been prepared. Of these, forty-three took the Certificate in Nursing Administration and sixty-nine took the Certificate in Nursing Education. A survey carried out by the unit towards the end of 1970 showed that seventy-two of the graduates had remained in their territories, even though a large number of them were still in positions they had occupied before they took the courses. In 1970 agreement was reached at the Caribbean health ministers' conference for the programme to be taken over by the governments of the region and UWI.[3]

This, then, was the state of events with regard to the ANEU when Mary took over as director. After the excitement over her appointment had calmed down, she set to work relentlessly in three roles in three pivotal organizations: as director of the ANEU; as a member of the executive of the NAJ, her professional organization; and as a representative of NAJ on the Nursing Council, the registration body for the profession. Her purpose was to bring about changes that would improve the standards and status of the nursing profession. Her goal was to promote nursing in the Caribbean. It was no longer to be seen as the poor sister of the medical profession. The public began to hear more about the profession and to see action on the part of nurses. The fact that she was the first West Indian nurse to have obtained a doctorate was also a selling point for nursing. She became a role model for younger nurses entering the field as the ANEU provided opportunity for advancement. It was only fitting that she would be among those honoured in Jamaica's national honours and awards, another first when, in 1974, she received the Order of Distinction, Commander Class (CD), for services to the nursing profession. She was described as a "very talented and dedicated leader", who had

> prepared herself over many years for her leadership role in this field, not only in the educational aspect but in administration and supervision in hospitals as well as Public Health Services. She has also been involved in research in nursing with special emphasis on planned programmes to enhance and further the standard of Nursing in the Caribbean region. She has given exemplary service in her chosen career, not only in Jamaica but also at the international level.[4]

As director of the ANEU, Mary fulfilled three roles: administrator, teacher and mentor. Generally speaking, administration and teaching are expectations of the university while the latter, arguably, is usually personal.

Administrator and Researcher

Mary's appointment coincided with the start of the second five-year period of the ANEU, during which it was expected that adequate physical facilities would be identified, the certificate curriculum enriched and expanded, and the Bachelor of Science degree course introduced. These were the major objectives. For the next five years, innumerable efforts were made by Mary and her faculty to obtain capital funding for a building, or even a part of a building, to house the unit. Contacts were made with government representatives, foundations, trust companies and other sources of funds. Explorations included local, regional and international agencies with no success. Reports to this effect were forwarded to successive conferences of health ministers, with the reminder that without adequate physical facilities there could be no appreciable expansion of the certificate programme nor implementation of the Bachelor of Science in Nursing degree programme. Finally, at their 1974 meeting, Caribbean health ministers requested that the CARICOM Secretariat seek external aid in the form of capital expenditure for the erection of a building for the ANEU. A resolution passed at the 1975 meeting requested the secretary general to continue to pursue efforts to this end. As a result, and in a collaborative effort between UWI and the secretariat, provision for physical facilities for the unit was made in an application to the European Development Fund in 1975.

At the end of 1971, as a prelude to the updating and enrichment of the curriculum, Mary conducted a follow-up study of ANEU graduates at the end of 1971. The study sought to find from past students, their supervisors and other important agencies the extent to which the certificate programme prepared graduates for effective performance in the territories and the attrition rate among graduates. Suggestions were requested for changes in the curriculum to make it more relevant to local needs. During the study Mary paid visits, partially funded by PAHO/WHO, to the larger territories and the others were contacted by mail. The results indicated that the graduates were performing satisfactorily, excellently in some cases, in middle-level teaching and administrative positions throughout the region. Many were occupying top level positions, beyond the expectations of the certificate programme, and were doing so with distinction. The attrition rate continued to be close to zero.

Of 112 graduates at that point in time, 105 were reported to be at their assigned jobs; 3 had stopped working temporarily for family reasons; 2 were away (probably overseas) on medical grounds; and the remaining 2 were pursuing studies in the United States. With regard to curriculum changes, suggestions were that more content in professional nursing and general health issues be included; more intensive field practice in both teaching and administration be given; and more assistance by the unit be given to students to help them with English and sociology courses. The need to start the degree programme and to assist in upgrading the skills of senior nurses to enable them to gain entry to the university were also stressed.

Based on these responses, the faculty undertook a major revision of the curriculum in 1972 and administrative changes were also implemented. New and more advanced content in nursing and health were included, as well as the development of a research methodology course. Faculty members were assigned specific responsibilities for groups of students, including the monitoring of courses given in other faculties or departments of the university with a view to providing supportive tutorials for students. Annual evaluation of all ANEU courses by students and faculty were also instituted on a formal basis and the results were to be shared with lecturers in other faculties or departments as necessary. Over the years, minor curricular changes emanated from these yearly evaluations. The changes in the curriculum over those five years proved to be beneficial to student performance in university examinations. The success rate among candidates rose from 50 percent during the initial five years of the ANEU to 80 percent after Mary had taken over and instituted these changes.

Yet another innovation arising out of the 1971 survey was the introduction of fieldwork to the eastern Caribbean islands. Mary's visits for evaluation of the programme showed her the need for more Caribbean nurses to benefit from the programmes of the ANEU in nontraditional ways. It was decided to hold part of the summer practicum in administration and teaching in selected territories outside Jamaica, with each group of students accompanied by a faculty member from ANEU. A proposal to have twenty-eight ANEU students do three weeks of their practicum in three territories – Barbados, Dominica, Trinidad and Tobago – was drawn up and submitted to PAHO/WHO and the territorial governments for shared funding.

PAHO and the governments concerned readily accepted the innovative proposal and the fieldwork went ahead as planned. The project continued for two more years, but after 1974 it was cancelled for lack of financial support. This development caused much disappointment to all parties, particularly as the yearly evaluations of the project had been very positive.

During 1975 the need for a second five-year comprehensive evaluation of the ANEU was under consideration, although not all the recommendations of the first evaluation of the unit had been fully implemented. The evaluation was to include a follow-up study of graduates' performance on the job over the last five years.

During this second five-year period, the proposal for a Bachelor of Science degree in nursing was further elaborated and presented at successive meetings of Caribbean health ministers. The health ministers were supplied with data on a ten-year projection of nursing education needs in each territory, including the financial implications, and had endorsed the continuation of the certificate programme with increased enrolment. They had also approved the introduction of the two-year programme leading to the Bachelor of Science in Nursing and committed themselves to meeting subsequent increases in recurrent costs.

The Bachelor of Science in Nursing programme was still not operational by 1976, due, among other things, to the lack of physical facilities. Enrolment had increased to thirty-six candidates in the certificate programme, but this was the absolute maximum since students were overcrowded in one classroom which also served as the library at the UHWI. There were increased efforts by all concerned at UWI to try to find alternative accommodation for the ANEU and eventually space was provided in the Postgraduate Medical Education Building of the Faculty of Medicine. The ANEU was temporarily relocated there on 1 January 1977 and enjoyed far more adequate space and facilities. Although this change in the status of the unit was temporary, Mary actively pursued the phased implementation of the Bachelor of Science in Nursing degree programme. There was now office accommodation for one more full-time tutor and shared classroom space was available within the Faculty of Medicine. Her diligence and persistence continued unabated.

Mary updated the degree proposal and submitted it to the Medical Faculty Board in March 1977 for its final approval and subsequent channelling through the relevant university committees. Her aim was to have the programme ready for the 1978/79 academic year. She had argued that any delay in implementing the programme would be potentially disastrous for UWI, as it was three years since the health ministers had committed their governments to the support of the programme on the basis of demonstrated need. She pointed out that although the ANEU was still without a permanent home, its faculty members were aware of the fact that programmes could not always wait for buildings. More importantly, she asserted that they wished to demonstrate the seriousness which they attached to the commitments given by the regional governments.

There were many valid and strong arguments for expediting the introduction of the Bachelor of Science in Nursing programme. In 1975 the Government of the Bahamas had withdrawn its financial support of the ANEU. The College of the Bahamas was newly opened and nursing was to be transferred to that setting. Consequently, more nurse tutors with a first degree were needed and the Bahamian government turned to the United States for assistance. An arrangement had been made with a university in Florida whereby Bahamian nurses could obtain a bachelor's degree on relatively easy terms. Transcripts for all eight of the past Bahamian students had been requested from the ANEU. Trinidad and Tobago had taken a decision to start their own Bachelor of Science in Nursing programme, but this programme never materialized. That territory had sent the second largest number of candidates to the ANEU, thirty-five, including the present class. The Regional Project for the Education and Training of Allied Health Personnel contemplated starting a multidisciplinary post-basic programme under the auspices of the United Nations Development Project and, since the bulk of its intended candidates would be nurses, the ANEU had proposed to the project management that the ANEU programme be used as the prototype for that project. The proposal, aimed at minimizing duplication and fragmentation, was accepted. Mary further argued that failure to initiate the degree programme could have far-reaching implications for the university, in general, and the unit, in particular. She observed that over the years, the graduates had grown tired of waiting for the start of the degree programme, and had gone to universities abroad and in the region to pursue degree courses. Since nursing degrees were not available in the region, these nurses had to study in other disciplines and very often, on graduation, they were lost to nursing. This sorry state of affairs was one that the Caribbean could ill afford.

Mary buttressed these arguments with yet further data regarding the Regional Nursing Body which had recommended that nursing education be conducted under the auspices of institutions in which education, not service, was the primary purpose. This significant recommendation had also been accepted by the Conference of Caribbean Ministers of Health in July 1975 in Montserrat. Mary's final argument was that, given the university's approval of the proposal without major modifications, it was estimated that about 120 past students of the ANEU would be eligible for admission to the programme on the basis of credit. This suggested that even with no change in the eligibility rate of future advanced nursing education students, a post-basic degree programme at the UWI could be supported within the region indefinitely.[5]

The NAJ also lobbied to get the programme started by writing to the minister of health urging financial commitment to start the programme in October 1978. Finally, after many years of planning and countless presentations, the proposal to start the degree programme received final approval by the University Academic Committee at its Mona meeting in March 1978. The inaugural class was set for October 1978. With this date in mind, Mary wrote to the permanent secretaries in the ministries of health of the various territories, with copies to the principal nursing officers, informing them of the eligibility of past students who had taken the certificate programme and had achieved at least a 'B' average in the three major courses. To expedite matters, a list of the names of all eligible candidates were included. They were entitled to receive full credit for one calendar year towards the degree programme.

Mary asked for responses from the ministries on a number of points in order to have an indication of the number of students who would be planning to enter the first class. Since most of the nurses were employees of the government through the Ministry of Health, their availability was fully dependent on whether or not the ministry would sponsor their attendance at the university. It was not only prudent but essential that Mary should have all that data readily available. Further, this was July 1978 and the degree programme was due to commence in October. A memorandum dated 17 July 1978 that Mary sent to Vice Chancellor Aston Preston, not only kept the senior administration of the university informed but indirectly urged them to take action with regard to funding the programme through the University Grants Committee. Copies of that memo and attachments were sent to all relevant senior personnel within the university.[6] A Bachelor of Science degree, with a major in nursing, was eventually introduced in October 1983 with thirteen students from three territories (Bahamas, Belize and Jamaica).

Her many accomplishments in Jamaica and the Caribbean did not go unrecognized by her alma mater in the United States. In 1981 the Nursing Education Alumni Association Award, from Teachers' College, Columbia University, was bestowed on her for distinguished achievement in the administration of nursing.

Mary's role as an administrator would not be complete without an exploration of her relationships with those to whom she reported and vice versa. The ANEU, as a part of the Department of Social and Preventive Medicine, was directly accountable to the head of that department; consequently Mary reported to Dr Kenneth Standard (now Sir Kenneth). His leadership style is best exemplified by his words and his actions. Tall, slender, and gentle in manner, Sir Kenneth has now retired but still visits the department on a weekly basis. He said that from the outset of Mary's appointment to the position of director of the unit, he had written to her in Geneva indicating that she had free rein to run the unit " 'as a department and I will only interfere as far as you want me to or ask me'. She had her own budget and she had her own programme . . . No one interfered, not even the chairman of the committee. So I wanted to reassure her . . . I give free rein because I take it that if people are happy in doing what they are doing, they will go beyond the normal bounds of duty and there are many ways of achieving some objectives . . . I thought it was even more important with the nurses because traditionally or historically, it was said that doctors thought they were this and that and kept back nurses. So they were coming into their own."[7]

Dr Standard and Mary attended many conferences together, including the conferences of ministers of health, where they were observers. He depicted her as "a person who couldn't suffer fools gladly. And sometimes her diplomatic tact might not have been the best. But I understood Mary and as time went on I understood the reasons for her attitude as she was always fighting for something for the nurses . . . She was anxious to get the best that she could for nurses and get it quickly." He continued, carefully, suggesting that she was really misunderstood: "As we conversed I saw the difficulty she had and the problems . . . that Mary projected was, one would say, justified or the problems she had as a youngster coming up . . . she did not have it easy – might have had some injustices meted out to her from time to time . . . And what has been interpreted as being difficult is because she's accustomed to fighting for everything." He credited her with establishing bridges of understanding between the profession and the community through the courses, students and the various islands.

A faculty member, Mary Grant, commented that "the thing I remember most in working with Dr Seivwright is that she was a very thorough person. Thorough and almost to the point of being a perfectionist . . . Because of her being so meticulous about many things, her administrative style was more autocratic . . . Everything had to be approved by Dr Seivwright. She spoke very elegantly, and wrote extremely well. Her documentation was above reproach . . . She did not tolerate any, what we might call, slackness . . . She was very demanding but in writing our evaluations, I found that she was very fair. She gave you credit where credit was due. Very, very fair. She was very honest. She'd listen to you if you had any ideas . . . but she basically ruled the roost. She had regular meetings with the staff . . . so everybody knew what was happening . . . I appreciated that . . . Dr Seivwright should be recognized as one of those stalwarts in nursing because she devoted so much of her time and energy in trying to get things for nursing."[8]

Enid Lawrence, who worked closely with her for many years, made a similar observation that regardless of her approach her objectives were to improve the nursing profession and to help nurses move ahead.

Mary Seivwright Research Day

The year 1989 marked the inauguration of the Mary Seivwright Day, instituted by the ANEU in honour of Mary. In 1990 this celebration was combined with the first annual nursing research conference and is now the Annual Nursing Research Conference and Mary Seivwright Day. It was acknowledged that research was her particular scholarly and academic endeavour. Further, she was lauded for her commitment to the purpose of instilling and inspiring the research skills of nurses. Syringa Marshall-Burnett, current director of the ANEU, now a department, noted that "Dr Seivwright has a passion for research. She has really worked overtime to pass on her enthusiasm for the subject and the work." To that end she strengthened the curriculum with an introductory research course which she taught, guiding nurses in their first attempts at research. Moreover, in addition to urging nurses to undertake serious investigations of suitable topics that were essentially nursing in nature, she sought to have nurses strengthen their intuitive and traditional practice with scientific study. They were encouraged to examine problems affecting the lives of ordinary people over which nurses could have some influence, for example, teenage pregnancy.

A DREAM COME TRUE

Mary had long dreamed that the ANEU would one day be granted departmental status within the Faculty of Medical Sciences and so become the main centre of higher education for nurses in the region. She envisioned post-basic as well as basic courses being offered and faculty being involved on the Mona campus and in non-campus territories throughout the region. She also ardently wanted the existing Faculty of Medical Sciences to be replaced by a Faculty of Health Sciences, with the proposed Department of Nursing as part of it. A Faculty of Health Sciences would include all the health disciplines requiring professional preparation, and possibly make a reality of the common wish for a health team.[9]

This notion of complementary and equal partnership of the health care team has been the Achilles' heel of nursing internationally. It was a bold and far-reaching vision for nursing in Jamaica in the 1970s. Even in North America, few schools of nursing in universities could lay claim to such equality. Invariably, the majority were 'under' a Faculty of Medicine or some other faculty. Although in recent times there is a Faculty of Health Sciences and nursing is independent as a department, or a school, the administration often includes a 'head' of health sciences who almost invariably is a male and a physician. Mary Seivwright's concept was truly visionary. Given the domination of gender and status in medicine and nursing in Jamaica at that time, when nursing was struggling to get a foothold in the university at the bachelor degree level, the prescience of her views becomes more remarkable.

The struggle for the ANEU to be recognized as a department had continued unsuccessfully as nursing had to compete with other units that also sought departmental status within the university body. Eventually the unit gained departmental status in 1991, some years after Mary's retirement, but her doggedness and determination had made her dream a reality after she had passed the mantle on to her equally determined and powerful successor, Syringa Marshall-Burnett.

The Nurse Practitioner Programme

A further development within the ANEU while Mary was the director was the Nurse Practitioner Programme. An innovative concept when it was first discussed in the early 1970s, it became one of the most successful initiatives of the unit. Today it remains a central programme for West Indian territories, administered by the Department of Advanced Nursing Education (DANE).

The notion of a nurse practitioner programme started among leaders of the NAJ in late 1971 to early 1972, while they were writing the NAJ's position paper on nursing in Jamaica. That exercise provided an excellent opportunity for senior nurses with overseas experience to exchange ideas on trends and issues in nursing. Mary was the chairperson of the Position Paper Working Party, and she and her colleagues shared information on the worldwide trend towards expanding the role of the nurse in the delivery of health care. Of particular interest to the group was the North American model that included the nurse practitioner. It appeared to have special relevance to the Jamaican situation. In anticipation of such a development, the position paper included the statement that "Nurses who, in addition to or instead of their normal nursing functions, have to provide health care of a medical nature must receive legal protection as well as additional compensation."[10]

NAJ members were excited about the possibility of such a programme for Jamaica and constantly talked about it among themselves and with all who would listen, including two former ministers of health. At last, on the evening of 10 January 1973, Mary, in her role as director of ANEU, received a phone call from Dr Ragbeer, dean of the Faculty of Medicine, inviting her to a meeting that same night at the home of Dr Mavis Gilmour, the then parliamentary secretary in the Ministry of Health. The intent of the meeting was to discuss how the UWI Faculty of Medicine could assist in the training of a "nurse-functionary" (no title had yet been decided) who would "extend the arm" of doctors and relieve them of some routine tasks. Dr Ragbeer went on to say that, knowing how strongly Mary felt about nursing matters, he was taking it upon himself to invite her to the meeting and he wondered whether she would accept the invitation under those conditions. She accepted the invitation with great alacrity.

Obviously, Mary had already established a reputation as a strong advocate for nursing and the importance of nursing input from the beginning of the decision-making process. Mary was the only nurse present at that exploratory meeting; all other members were from the Faculty of Medicine. During the discussions, Dr Gilmour tried in vain to prevent participants from attaching a title to this intended 'functionary'. Terms such as 'medical assistant', 'clinical assistant', and 'medex', were bandied about. Mary's contributions to the list were 'nurse practitioner' and 'nurse clinician'. Most of those present at that first meeting saw this 'functionary' as being hospital-based, working 'under the eye' of a doctor. Mary was asked if the ANEU would be interested in participating in such a training programme. Her initial response was in the negative as she explained that the unit would not be prepared to take senior professional nurses, give them additional preparation, and then place them under the supervision of another health care profession. All those at the meeting agreed that these 'functionaries' should be trained to work in paediatrics, general practice, especially chronic diseases, and psychiatry.

Mary recalled that after the meeting a member of the group suggested that she had perhaps made a tactical mistake in her stand against the participation of the unit in the programme. She agreed that his point was well taken but she felt that as a matter of principle and in her capacity as director of the ANEU she could not take any other position. However, she continued, within a few days she would be wearing another hat as president of NAJ and what she expected to say there would differ substantially. This was Mary's forte: using her political skills and having the wisdom to know when to change hats in order to use the power of the group, her professional organization, to further the goals of nursing.

A second exploratory meeting was called by Dr Gilmour on 8 March 1973 to review reports submitted by the select committees. Soon other individuals and groups, such as the NAJ and the Medical Association of Jamaica (MAJ), became involved in discussions about the start of such a programme. In June a special meeting was called by NAJ in order to discuss the position of the association on a nurse practitioner programme for Jamaica. The Nurse Practitioner Committee then formed was charged with the responsibility of developing a proposal for submission to the Ministry of Health at the earliest possible date. In September 1974 the NAJ proposal for the establishment of the Nurse Practitioner Programme was submitted to the Ministry of Health and accepted with enthusiasm by the then minister of health, Dr Ken McNeill, and the government. The proposal was also endorsed and fully supported by the MAJ and it formed the basis for the development of the programme. Implementation, however, was another matter. Changes in senior government ministry personnel delayed progress.

Project HOPE (Health Opportunities for People Everywhere) had been involved with the programme from the beginning. In February 1977 Dr Robert Chamblin, a consultant with Project HOPE, wrote to Dr Henry Clark, Jr, director of Project HOPE, noting that everyone concerned agreed that the Nurse Practitioner Programme was of high priority and needed to get started as soon as possible. He added that it was an exciting project that would have considerable impact on the health services of Jamaica and on other Caribbean countries as well. Among his recommendations was the need to have the minister of health make a definite budget commitment as soon as possible to aid in recruitment for those interested in serving as counterparts to the faculty provided by Project HOPE. It was further recommended that the programme should start after 1 July 1977.[11]

Mary credited the parliamentary secretary, Dr Winston Davidson, with making the Nurse Practitioner Programme become a reality through his professional commitment and political courage. She claimed that he had made what was beginning to look like an administrative impossibility happen, as on the date recommended, the Nurse Practitioner Programme began with the registration of twenty-five students, of whom eighteen were in the Family Nurse Practitioner Programme and seven in the Nurse Paediatrician Programme. All those taking the course came from permanent positions with the Ministry of Health. They were drawn from hospitals, health centres and public health nursing posts scattered over eleven parishes. The majority of these women were married with families, so there was a great deal of sacrifice on their part.

The programme was one year in length, with a six-week core curriculum, for all students, consisting of general subjects such as sociology, introduction to research methods, nursing and related subjects, and common specialist topics such as health history and physical examination. These core activities were followed by a two-stranded specialist curriculum of eighteen weeks, consisting of courses relevant to those who were in the family or paediatrics stream. Following these six months of theoretical content with relevant clinical demonstrations, a six-month internship was carried out in two three-month phases. The first phase was carried out under intense guidance and supervision of clinical preceptors based in and around the corporate area. The second phase placed students at the location of their permanent work assignment, or as close to it as possible, and was carried out with less intense preceptorship. Throughout the programme, there was provision for periodic performance evaluations and feedback, all of which contributed to the final evaluation. Provision was also made for a total evaluation of all courses and revision of the curriculum prior to the subsequent intake of students.

The nurse practitioner was viewed as a senior professional who possessed the minimum qualifications of a registered nurse or midwife – in the case of men, acceptable suitable substitute post-basic preparation in lieu of midwifery – with at least five years of post-registration practice in a relevant clinical speciality, and who had completed an approved programme for the education or training of nurse practitioners in a selected clinical discipline. The nurse practitioner would provide in-depth nursing care and would assume agreed-upon, specific responsibilities and functions of a medical nature, acting independently with clear delegation of authority. Each nurse practitioner would work in consultation and collaboration with at least one licensed physician, regardless of the location of the physician. The nurse practitioner would also relate to and cooperate with other nursing colleagues and would be directly responsible to the employer or employer representative.

Mary contended that Jamaican nurses fitted neatly into such a framework as, traditionally, they had demonstrated that they were capable of expanding their role and had accepted responsibility for various aspects of health care beyond their responsibilities as nurses, without additional preparation, remuneration, recognition or legal protection. She pointed out that, given the increasing shortage of medical personnel to serve the majority of the Jamaican people, especially those in the rural and overpopulated areas and inner-city centres, it seemed logical that the country should turn to and adequately equip selected nurses to assume the expanded role. The nurse practitioner, she asserted, should not be viewed as a replacement for or a displacement of any other group of health care providers, but as a complement to the cadre of health professionals possessing the high-level clinical skills that were in critically short supply. Mary knew that the need for such a worker was clear.

The Joint Nurse Practitioner Advisory Committee was formed and became operational in early 1977. It was composed of representatives from the Ministry of Health, UWI, the NAJ, the MAJ, the nursing and medical councils, Project HOPE, and other invited participants. The committee advised on policy and other matters affecting implementation and monitoring of the project activities. An important subcommittee of that body was dealing with the legal aspects of the nurse practitioner: the development of legislation and regulations related to the prescribing of drugs and the role of the practitioners in death certification.[12]

Because the Nurse Practitioner Programme was a collaborative venture between the Ministry of Health and the Faculty of Medicine, UWI, this combination resulted in some administrative difficulties. Project HOPE and the Ministry of Health provided the personnel, trainers and their counterparts. The university was responsible for curricular activities through the faculty participation, drawing on the Department of Social and Preventive Medicine, of which the ANEU was a part, and the School of Education. Day-to-day administration fell on Mary as director of the ANEU and also the director of the Nurse Practitioner Programme. The programme was housed in the Ministry of Health at the Flamingo Complex on Half Way Tree Road, since there were no suitable facilities on or adjacent to the UWI campus. This created some logistic problems as the ministry had to provide assistance with certain aspects of administration; Mary functioned with some difficulty as the whole operation was not as smooth and efficient as she would have liked it to be.

In 1979 Mary approached Enid Lawrence, who was then head of the UHWI School of Nursing, to ask her if she would act as director of the Nurse Practitioner

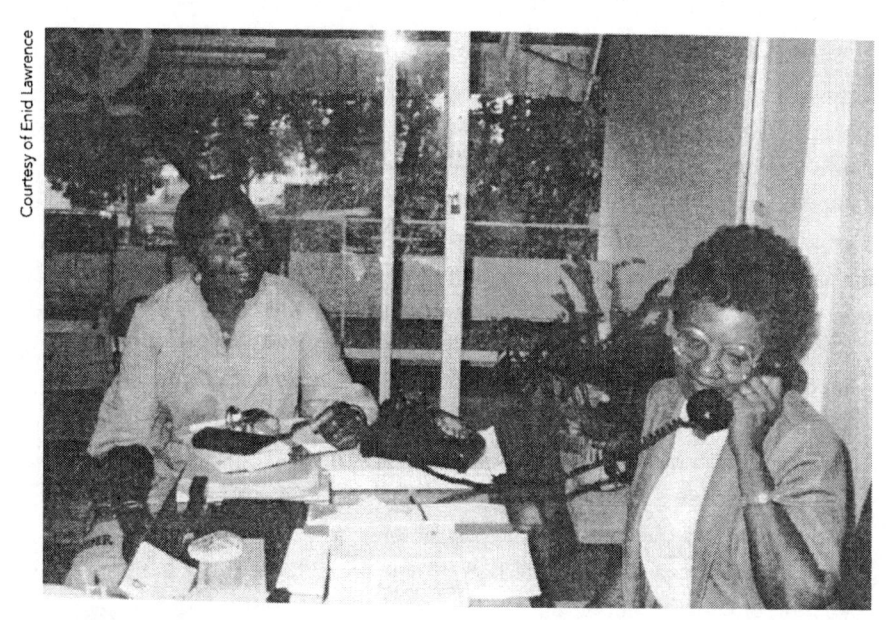

Mary Seivwright with Enid Lawrence, coordinator of the Nurse Practitioner Programme, in the coordinator's office, 1982

Programme for one year on secondment. Enid agreed to take the post and she eventually stayed on for five years. At the time of writing, the Ministry of Health now has responsibility for the day-to-day administration of the programme through a coordinator.

Enid remembered that long before the Nurse Practitioner Programme started, Mary had been concerned about nurses in the rural communities who were carrying out various activities and meeting the needs of the people without proper formal training or status. She saw the programme really as an extension of the nurses' skills. A continuing education component was incorporated into the programme soon after its inception. Some of the graduates were trained to become continuing education 'officers' and were sent to the various regions. All the practitioners within a region would meet once a month to review their 'cases' and hold seminars on important issues. Twice yearly, all the practitioners would meet in Kingston for a major seminar with a theme and special guest speakers. Enid emphasized that "it was Dr Mary's foresight in building a curriculum which ensured that a high standard of practice of the nurse practitioners would be maintained through continuing education and opportunities to improve their standard of practice at all times".

From the beginning, the programme had included nurses from Belize. Subsequently, nurses from the other West Indian territories had been admitted for training. Many of them went abroad to work as nurse practitioners and they were always welcome in all kinds of communities. Enid told an anecdote to illustrate the success of the programme and its impact in Jamaica. In one community, the doctor went in early and saw all his patients. When the nurse practitioner arrived, she always found a lot of patients waiting to see her. Finally, she discovered that after the patients had left the doctor, they went around to the back of the building and 'lined up' to see her. It turned out that the patients wanted to see the nurse practitioner because she spent time listening to and talking with them. The nurse practitioners also followed up on patients who, for one reason or another, did not keep their appointment at the clinics. A protocol manual, incorporating the basic medical conditions which a nurse practitioner frequently encountered and was able to diagnose and prescribe for, was designed.[13]

Enid pointed out that Mary had worked with the Nurse Practitioner Programme from its inception until her retirement and that it was to her credit that very high standards were always maintained. It was hardly surprising that in 1979 she received a special award for community service from the St Andrew Jaycees (of Jamaica).

Mary achieved much as an administrator and demanded excellence in the programmes under her administration. She demanded no less as a teacher.

Teacher and Mentor

Mary taught research methodology to students in the certificate and then the Bachelor of Science in Nursing courses as well as to the nurse practitioners. She profoundly believed in the importance of research in practice and in education. This strong conviction coupled with her demands for excellence gave her the reputation of being a formidable character. One of her colleagues, Lucy Flash O'Sullivan, president of the NAJ in 1973, preceding Mary's term of office, was a student in the ANEU. She told me that, with Mary, friendship and performance were two different things: "Fear was struck in the heart of all of us when Mary came into that room to teach her methodology." But she also noted that Mary knew the names of all her students and at the end of the class would give Lucy vegetables brought for her from Mary's property.

Another of Mary's students, Yvonne Young Reid, chief executive officer of the Spanish Town Hospital, reflected on her experiences and the lasting impact that Mary had made on her. She said that while many nurses had gone away and reached leadership positions in nursing, none had returned to Jamaica to create an awareness of leadership and the importance of research in the nursing profession. Mary had brought a dignity and a consciousness to nursing and to leadership in particular. All the students who came under her influence as a teacher had the undergirding of research. Indeed, her name became synonymous with research. Not only did she teach nursing research methodology but she also stretched students to their limits, and perhaps beyond in some cases. It was clear that she was a role model for many, not in her teaching approach but in her drive to have them be the best that they could be. Yvonne commented, "I think that she would be my mentor in terms of my thought process and aspirations as a leader. I do believe that she had a tremendous impact on me and I believe that where I am today, in part, has been stimulated by that early involvement with Mary Jane."[14]

Mary Seivwright was also a feminist in her own way. She shared many anecdotes with students about receiving 'put-downs' abroad, and using them as 'turn-arounds' that challenged her. These incidents made her determined to emerge as the person she was being made to feel, she could not become. She achieved that. She was proud to admit that she was from a poor background and had made it, and they could too. She stimulated them to greater heights. Self-improvement was her motto. Mary encouraged students to take a stand and express their opinions confidently and positively even if they were wrong, if they believed their opinions were right at the time. As more information became available, that stand might change. Yvonne credited Mary with teaching her that concept of decision making. Hermi Hewitt, a faculty member, concurred, "Students must have an opinion whether it is right or wrong and they were to defend their point of view . . . She was an exemplary person and her impression on every student is that she gave her all."[15]

Yvonne recounted an incident where, in her previous role as nursing director, responsible for secondary and tertiary care in the Ministry of Health, she was interviewing a nurse for a particular position. She was using an analytical approach in helping the nurse to decide the best course of action for her at that time. The nurse complimented her by commenting that she was just like Dr Seivwright.

Mary could be a great teacher in assisting students to analyse issues, but her approach left many in tears. It has been said that her autocratic style of teaching hindered the learning of some students. Nevertheless, she encouraged them to laugh at themselves and honestly admit that individuals had different teaching and learning styles, and that they were to be patient with one another – no doubt alluding to herself and her approach. Her drive, her direction, the intellectual process she used in terms of achieving and motivating others, and stimulating them to learn were what mattered to those like Yvonne. She said, "I don't think that . . . what was otherwise interpreted as her negative personality mattered too much to me, or even noticed by me, because I had fun going into Mary Jane's office to have discussions with her . . . and many of my colleagues passed through that year maybe just sitting before her just for the one time . . . at the discussion of our grades, and that was a pity because they never got to know her."

Mary very often used a combative, confrontational style or approach in her encounters with others, whether on committees, teaching, or as an administrator. Some were concerned that she was too forceful, too intimidating, while others felt she was like "a cold, scolding mother". Her admirers countered this with the fact that she had a noble objective – that she was singularly focused on moving nursing ahead at home and developing leaders who could 'stand up' internationally – but allowed that in achieving this she lost some in the process. This in no way diminished what many saw as her extraordinary gifts of zeal, enthusiasm, and keen analytical skills.

Another significant area in which Mary influenced her students was the importance of the individual as an agent of change and, even more important, the role of the nurse in policy making. She would share with her students knowledge about writing proposals and lobbying government alike, and also her own encounters with leaders of government throughout the Caribbean. Her experience exposed her students to a nursing leader who was intimately involved with the content and process of policy making in progress. They learned the importance of persistence and assertiveness in achieving goals. She told her students about one notable incident. Nursing was being discussed at a board meeting of UWI, and no representation from nursing had been invited. Mary dressed herself suitably for the occasion, entered the board meeting, introduced herself, apologized for the board not inviting her, sat down and made her contribution to what they were discussing about nursing. Needless to say, everyone, including the vice chancellor, was flabbergasted! These anecdotes left the students in awe of her. She had a biblical phrase, "Fully clothed and in your right mind", which was often quoted to alert them when taking a stand on nursing matters, to be appropriately attired and well-armed with the data. It was her strong belief that nurses needed to be proactive to ensure a better education for themselves and better standards of health care for the people. Marina Andrewin Staine proudly acknowledged the impact Mary had on her personally and professionally. She attributed Mary with being the key to opening her eyes to the whole domain of advanced nursing practice. "Accountability was the watchword – accountability for self, for nursing practice, and for what went on in one's country." Through Mary's influence she developed a philosophy of nursing, principles and values that served her in good stead not only in her practice but in her personal life.

Another former student, Pearlie Esteen, president of the NAJ in 1996, saw Mary as a perfectionist. She described Mary as being dynamic and one who "likes perfection . . . And so you will find that many of her students have gone to tears because of her perfectionism. She does not accept mediocrity . . . All her students have to perform. She aspires to get 'A' students."[16] Merel Hanson, retired principal nursing officer, also a former student, reiterated much of what others had said of her: Mary was a hard taskmaster and demanded perfection. "Some people are afraid of her, but I usually say her bark is more than her bite. When she is hard on you is that she wants you to perform at your best . . . She is somebody who crosses her t's and dots her i's . . . I have to give her credit for that. Because during my years at ICN, I was looked upon as the same sort of stickler for correctness . . . I used to say I was taught by Mary and I cannot do any better . . . once you train under her and decide that you will imitate her, you will arrive somewhere. I have Mary to thank for where I reached in nursing."[17]

THE NURSES' ASSOCIATION OF JAMAICA

Mary's contribution to her professional association, the NAJ, was awesome. She was president in 1974, 1975 and 1980. However, it was not the number of times that was significant, as many others had been elected three times, but it was her ceaseless manifold contributions that were daunting to many. As president she was very dynamic and very influential. She has been credited with putting Jamaican nurses on the map, locally, regionally and internationally. Her major contributions to the association centred around the socioeconomic welfare of nurses and their education for leadership roles. Here again, she took on the role of *de facto* teacher and mentor. She never lost touch with the association, even when she was not on the board or the executive. She was conscientious in her attendance at meetings and if she were unable to attend, she would call the association headquarters to find out what was happening.

Her health has been failing in recent years, but she still goes to the office occasionally to read the latest minutes. Pearlie Esteen spoke in admiration of Mary, describing her as a role model, while allowing that there were those who complained about "her mouth". She added, "And have no fear, she is still very articulate. She's very, very careful and very meticulous . . . she looks for every 'i' to be dotted and every 't' to be crossed and if it is not done, she'll say 'Pearlie, come on, we're an association, we're growing. What kind of nonsense is this? Get your officers to do better because these are for the records. We can't have this in an Association. No, we have to show that we are professionals and act accordingly.'

By 1971, shortly after she had been appointed director of the ANEU, Mary was on the executive of the NAJ. The association had for a long time expressed the need to provide more active leadership and direction for the improvement of nursing education and practice, and the socioeconomic conditions of nurses. At the second island conference of the NAJ in August 1971, which was also the occasion of their twenty-fifth anniversary, the members agreed that the association should put on record its position regarding nursing in Jamaica. Thus, at the first meeting of the new executive committee, held in September 1971, the decision was taken to assign to the Nursing Services Subcommittee of the NAJ the task of developing a position paper. The subcommittee assigned a working group the task of preparing the position paper articulating the NAJ's stand on matters affecting the nursing profession in Jamaica for presentation, discussion and adoption at their third island conference.

Enid Lawrence, head of the nursing school at the UWI Hospital was the president of the association, and had the opportunity to work closely with Mary on the development of this blueprint. One major objective of the NAJ was to give a vision of where nursing should be in terms of education, practice and socioeconomic matters. Mary provided dynamic leadership for this major initiative. Enid found the experience of working with Mary at the helm very challenging because of Mary's vision of bringing together senior nurses to make a contribution as to the direction nursing should go. The working party consisted of prominent leaders of nursing in the island, representing various areas of nursing. Among them were Leleka Champagnie, a former president of the association who was with the Ministry of Health; Gertrude Swaby, who was the editor of the nursing journal *Jamaican Nurse;* as well as the registrar of the Nursing Council, Julie Symes. Mary was the chairperson and the driving force in getting the position paper of the

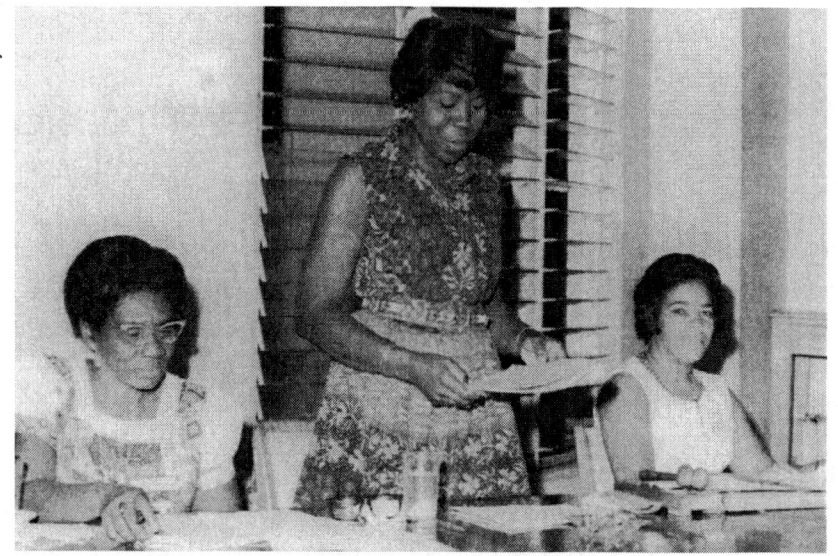

Lucy O'Sullivan (president of the Nurses' Association of Jamaica), Mary Seivwright and Iris Vassall-Bogues at the Nursing Education Seminar, 1973

working group published in a manual that was presented to and adopted by the NAJ membership at the third island conference and annual general meeting held in Port Maria in the following year. This manual eventually provided for years to come the guidelines for many changes within the profession.[18]

As president of the NAJ, Mary was instrumental in the formation of the association's credit union, and she was the first president of the union. The first members started out with a study club and rose from humble beginnings until the credit union now has over a thousand members. Another of her ideas was that the union should also serve the relatives and close friends of nurses, and this was reflected in the policies of the credit union.

She and her colleague Leleka Champagnie were among those who in the early days of the NAJ lobbied for the acquisition of the new premises at Trevennion Park Road, Kingston, where the association is currently housed. When the first headquarters of the NAJ (72 Arnold Road), which also housed the Nursing Council, became too small for a growing organization and was in need of expansion, Mary and Leleka spearheaded a proposal asking nurses to lend or give $100 each to aid in the expansion. However, it was not feasible to extend the existing building and the decision was taken to buy a property that could house the NAJ. The money contributed by the nurses and invested bought the premises at Trevennion Park Road, selected over other possible sites because of its central location. Syringa Marshall-Burnett was president of the NAJ at the time and the hostel is named after Leleka Champagnie. Leleka was then the nursing welfare officer in the Ministry of Health and saw clearly the need for a hostel to provide accommodation for nurses, particularly those who came from the rural areas to study in Kingston. Many nurses in the past had to defer taking courses for lack of accommodation. Leleka persisted in her efforts to make her idea for a hostel a reality. The association also wanted to be able to do something tangible for rural nurses on short-term courses and so the hostel was finally built. It can now accommodate thirty-two nurses and there is always full occupancy. There is also accommodation for a house mother and a hostel supervisor. Nurses from abroad could also stay there, but those outside the profession are discouraged. The new office building is also tenanted and the credit union rents space in the original building. These are sources of additional revenue for the NAJ, and so the whole organization is a viable economic venture. When the beginning of the NAJ is recalled, contained in a suitcase kept under Nita Barrow's bed, the achievement can be seen to be nothing less than amazing.

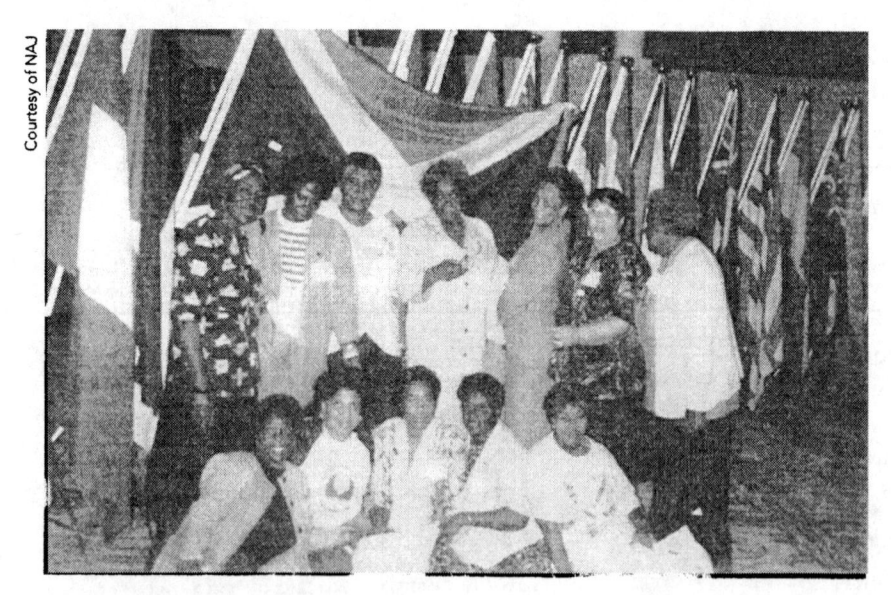

Standing at left, Mary Seivwright with the Jamaican registered nurses' delegation to the International Council of Nurses, Korea, 1989

While she was president in 1974, Mary nominated Merel Hanson for the position of secretary of the NAJ and became her mentor. Merel became actively involved in the association and held a variety of executive positions. She attended regional and international meetings and was eventually elected vice president in ICN, the only Caribbean nurse at that time to have reached that level. She proudly remarked, "I have [Mary] to thank for all this . . . because she would show you . . . she would tell you . . . she was a mentor to me. She supported you . . . Having seen that you are climbing, she gave you encouragement." Merel cited many examples of the support that Mary provided. It was not an easy role to be Mary's mentee, and many of them were afraid of her demand for excellence but they agreed that, in the final analysis, they all benefited from the experience.

The Road to Collective Bargaining

Mary continued her zest for nursing in yet another direction – the move toward the NAJ becoming the bargaining unit for all the nurses. Her impact on the socioeconomic condition of nurses was outstanding. In the 1970s, when Mary became active in the association, the momentum within the NAJ was high. There was a new sense of militancy among nurses and a readiness for change. A view of what was occurring in the society at large provides the background to this vitality.

In the mid 1960s emigration of nurses to North America approached alarming proportions. The major reasons were economic concerns and professional opportunities for advancement, while at the same time, there was a shortage of nurses in the United States and Canada. Many incentives were used to attract nurses. Recruiters from the United States visited the island to lure nurses away with a variety of attractive benefits, including opportunities for personal and professional advancement. Working conditions and salaries were the crux of the problem for all Jamaican nurses, whether members of the NAJ or not. Compounding the situation was the revelation that the government was planning to recruit British-trained nurses at 'higher salaries' to replace those who were leaving, but there was no indication that Jamaican nurses could expect better remuneration. A further complication was that nurses, as a body, had no professional representation to negotiate with the government. Apart from the nurses working at the UWI Hospital, almost all Jamaican nurses are employees of the government and consequently civil servants. All negotiations regarding working conditions, salaries or any other grievances had to be channelled through the Civil Service Association.

The nurses had never been happy with this arrangement. They believed that their concerns were not properly addressed by union representatives who had little or no understanding of the health field. Further, nurses were few in number compared to clerical workers who comprised 90 percent of government employees. In addition, one of the trade unions was attempting to infiltrate the nursing profession, claiming representational rights for all nurses because of the NAJ's brief through the Civil Service Association. This concern led to increased militancy on the part of the nurses because they wished to prevent the trade union speaking on their behalf.

Consequently, the nurses began to agitate for their own bargaining unit. However, no attention was paid to their grievances, even in the face of an islandwide demonstration in the mid 1960s when the nurses wore black sashes. The protest was orchestrated by the NAJ to bring attention to the need for better conditions. The Ministry of Health responded with the same approach that their colonial masters had used in the past by launching an investigation into the conditions of nursing service and training in the island. Colonialism had replicated itself. For, as it was so aptly put, "Independent Jamaica, despite the formal transfer of sovereignty, remained at heart a society still shaped by the colonial heritage."[19]

When Mary became president of the NAJ in 1974, she took up the cause with passion. She worked closely with Leleka, who by then had been hired by the association to be their full-time economic welfare officer, with the purpose of improving working conditions for nurses. Several delegations went to the Ministry of Health to plead their cause. Eventually, their persistence was rewarded. The minister of health indicated to Mary and her delegation that if they could enrol 80 percent of the nurses in Jamaica in the association, the ministry would consider bargaining rights. That was all Mary and Leleka needed to mount a vigorous campaign. They travelled around the island, talking to nurses and encouraging them to join the association and outlining the benefits that they would reap. While they journeyed across the island on their recruiting drive, together with Lucy Flash O'Sullivan, they created a song called the NAJ theme song, sung to the tune of "John Brown's Body". Needless to say, the association got the desired 80 percent membership.

One of the many initiatives generated by Mary and Leleka was a brief, written by Mary, to present to hearings of the Industrial Disputes Tribunal (IDT) in 1975. The NAJ had identified an anomaly between the paraprofessional and professional nursing groups in terms of salary and sought redress. The matter was referred to

An Extraordinary Woman

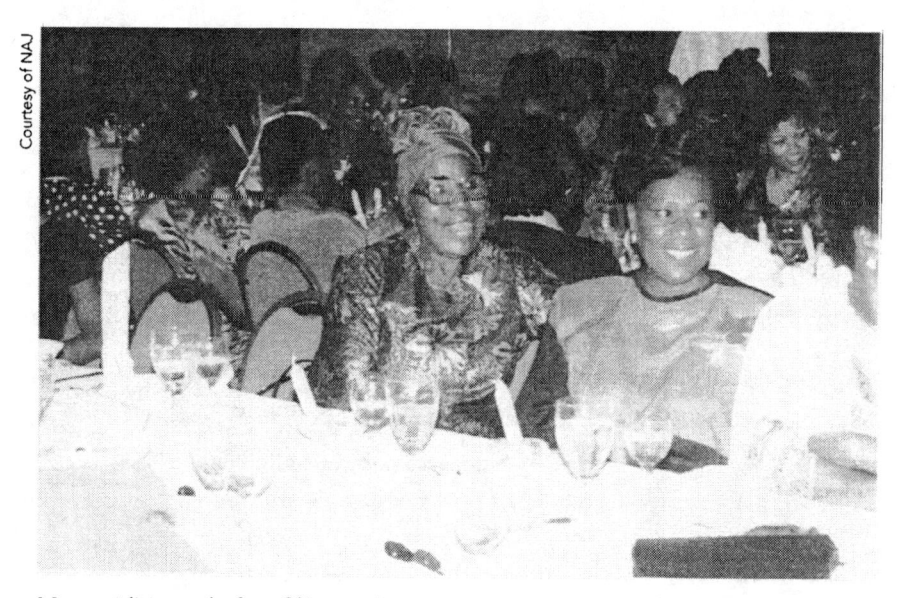

Mary socializing at the forty-fifth annual general meeting of the Nurses' Association of Jamaica, Mallards Beach Hotel, Ocho Rios, Jamaica, 1991

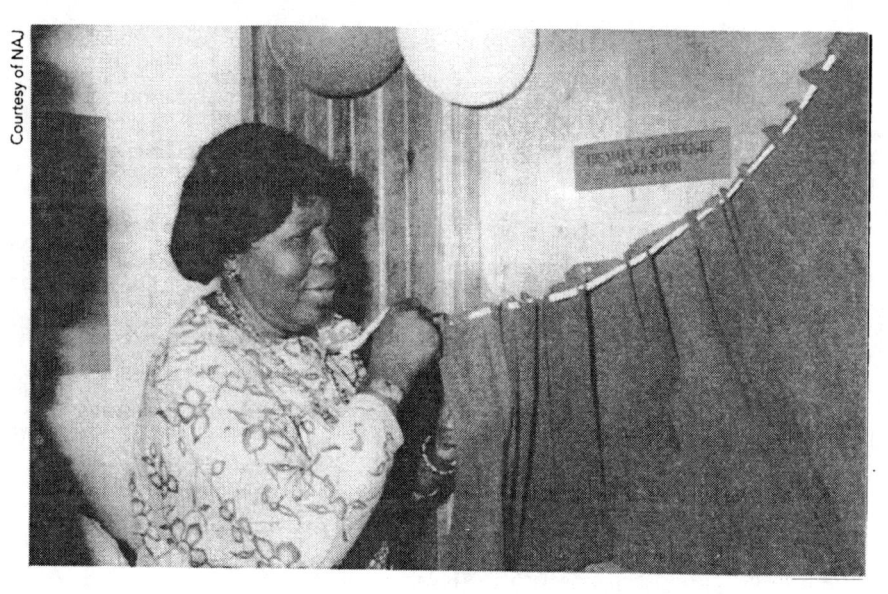

Mary unveiling the plaque in her honour, at the Nurses' Association of Jamaica boardroom, Kingston, 1995

the IDT. The nurses enlisted a lawyer to refine the legal aspects of their submission to the tribunal but there was no success that year. By the following year, however, a better differential was created by the government. Further developments that the nurses achieved through negotiations with government under Mary's guidance were an examination of the working week, modification of the hours of work, and compensation for overtime and for uniforms. Nurses with post-basic preparation and experience were rewarded financially, if not promoted, and promotions were not only by seniority as had previously been the practice. A major achievement was that nurses were to be paid sessional rates for every additional four hours and for being 'on call', as were the doctors. Prior to that, nurses were frequently 'on call', because of shortage of staff, without being paid for this or for any overtime. This could happen on weekdays and weekends, including public holidays. Many leaders in the profession had argued vigorously in the past for those improvements but it took Mary to make them a reality. Mary's success was attributed to her assertiveness and confidence in dealing with the minister as an equal because of her higher degrees and her dogged persistence.

Mary is further credited with changes in the constitution of the association. Life membership and honorary life membership were introduced, with criteria for each category. To qualify for life membership, a nurse would pay a prescribed fee but should also have given outstanding service to the association in order to be considered for the honour. Honorary life membership was an honour bestowed on a nurse after having given outstanding service to the association. Her other major contribution within the NAJ was orchestrating the use of the professional body as a vehicle to get the Nurse Practitioner Programme implemented and funded by government.

The association paid tribute to her by naming their boardroom in her honour in May 1995. Because of her dynamism at meetings it was felt that the boardroom should be named after her. One story told is of Mary's militancy at a board meeting when she became so incensed that she broke the gavel! The address delivered by Merel Hanson on that occasion cited a number of firsts that Mary had accomplished as a black woman, a Jamaican nurse, and a Caribbean nurse. Among her many accolades, Merel noted:

the negotiator, the consultant, the mentor, the friend, the counsellor, the loud 'barker' but 'soft biter'. For, excellence, the nurse who has a motivating word – solidarity . . . The Board room of the Nurses Association of Jamaica (NAJ) with the chief seat held by Mary Jane Seivwright has been the place where many a plan was conceived, discussed, implemented and evaluated for the improvement of nursing and health care and for the socioeconomic welfare of nurses . . .

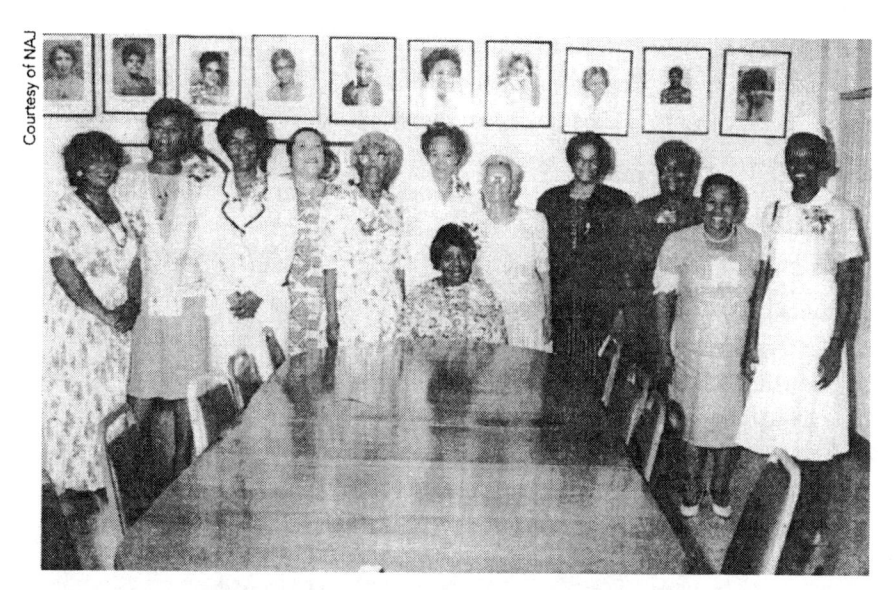

Mary with past presidents and honoured nurses at the naming of the Nurses' Association of Jamaica boardroom in her honour, Kingston, 1995. From left to right, Perlie Esteen, Janet Coorefarr (nurse of the year), Pat Ivers, Syringa Marshall-Burnett, Lucille Lindsay, Merel Hanson, Cynthia Vernon, Lucy O'Sullivan, Leleka Champagnie, Carmen Brooks, and Marlene Dixon (nursing student of the year)

May she continue to influence us by her words and actions and the feeling of her presence as we meet in this conference room; and may those after us who may not meet her be conscious of the work and worth of this great Jamaican through their entry in this Boardroom.[20]

THE NURSING COUNCIL

The final organization in the trio of Mary's selfless devotion was the Nursing Council. From November 1972 to February 1993 Mary was a member of the council as a representative of the NAJ. In that role, she provided guidance and direction to bring about changes in the functioning of the Nursing Council and in many of its activities. It was quite an exercise for council members when Mary came to meetings. Because of her insistence on accuracy, it sometimes took up to two hours to amend the minutes. Members learned a lot about parliamentary procedure for meetings as she ensured that rules were enforced and maintained, and that records were correct so that new members coming along would learn how to follow them. While she was on the Nursing Council, members also had the opportunity to gain experience and knowledge about evaluating schools of nursing. During her stewardship, Excelsior Community College and the West Indies College (which was started by the Seventh Day Adventist Church), among others, were evaluated. Mary's educational expertise in that realm was deemed extremely useful as many of the leaders did not have the kind of exposure that she had. It was a learning experience for many. One outstanding change was that minimum uniform standards were set for the entry of students into nursing schools in the island. Prior to that, each nursing school had its own standards.

Theresa Boyne admitted that she learned a tremendous amount from Mary. When Theresa was appointed registrar of the Nursing Council in 1984, Mary was already a member of the council and, in Theresa's words, "She was a dedicated nurse. In addition to that, she does not settle for mediocrity. Dr Mary is excellence. Excellence is her watchword. Anything she is doing it must be well done. Perfection almost. And she expects the same of anybody else, who worked with her . . . and she [has] lived this right through her life."[21] To illustrate the importance Mary paid to the affairs of the Nursing Council, Theresa said that when Mary got her new diary for the year, she would not only mark on her calendar the dates for every council meeting but also block in the entire day so that she would have no other appointment for that day. She further insisted that all members and the staff did likewise. It is interesting to note that Mary never assumed the chair of council. She was adamant about this because she preferred to be a member and could make the greatest impact by challenging all the items that came to the floor. She was always well-prepared for meetings so that no item on the agenda took her by surprise nor was she unable to contribute to any item.

One of her outstanding achievements during her two decades with the council was spearheading the development of a policy for nurses covering their 'delegated function' of vena puncture. In Jamaica nurses are called upon almost daily to perform intravenous drug therapy, blood transfusions and similar procedures. It was becoming increasingly common for the physicians to turn this over to the nurses to avoid having to work evenings or weekends. A working group was set up with key nursing personnel from the Ministry of Health, the heads of nursing schools, matrons of the teaching hospitals and midwifery schools under Mary's tutelage and guidance, to develop a policy covering vena puncture by nurses. The group worked assiduously for many years in refining the policy, principles and procedures, and in designing a formal training course that included an evaluative component for both the course and its graduates. The training programme will ultimately be implemented as the policy was finally approved in 1996, almost ten years after its initial submission. In the meantime, the nurses will, as before, continue to carry out vena puncture. The steadfastness of the nurses in pursuing this policy is to be admired. Theresa noted that "Mary was the backbone to all this policy development . . . She was the guiding light behind it all."

Another major contribution attributed to Mary was the idea of the biennial renewal of the licence to practise by registered nurses. The Nursing Council, along with the NAJ, had initially been working on the idea of a triennial renewal of licence for many years, because nurses are registered for life. However, when Mary became a member of council she suggested changing it to a biennial renewal. Conditions have been set for biennial renewal, which included, after many revisions, sixty hours of continuing education over the two years. The highly centralized nature of nursing means that the minister of health must approve a proposal before it can go to the legislature. While the nurses have been commended for moving ahead in attempting to make keeping abreast of knowledge and skills a prerequisite for continued registration, to date that initiative was still in abeyance. A major concern appears to have been the cost of continuing education for nurses. Government would have to pay staff attending courses and seminars and also pay for their temporary replacements. With regard to advanced nursing practice, there was an apparent stalemate between nurse anaesthetists who wanted to have a separate register from nurse practitioners. Little advance has been made on that front. However, the Nursing Council is now working on a revised proposal for a separate register for nurses in advanced practice that would cover the various categories. That concept appeared to be more conciliatory and could perhaps be more acceptable to nurse anaesthetists.

On a smaller scale, prior to her leaving the council, Mary did a mini research project for the council on why young people did not choose nursing as a career. This was a challenge to the Ministry of Health, which argued that the entrance requirement of four O-level courses was a deterrent. The report was never completed because of Mary's failing eyesight. However, her interim findings submitted to the minister of health indicated that the poor image of nursing, poor working conditions and low salaries were the main reasons for low recruitment into the profession and not the entrance requirements. The latter has been the standard argument put forth by governments universally. They downgraded the importance of educated nurses, primarily female. This gender bias and power attitude have held true internationally in the growth and development of the profession. In North America, the struggle to get higher educational requirements for nurses as entry into the profession, or to obtain a university education for nurses, has been met with resistance from both the government and the medical profession, and even within the profession itself. The struggle of nurses in Jamaica was similar to their counterparts elsewhere, only at a different point in time.

Mary was nominated on more than one occasion by the Nursing Council to receive the Order of Jamaica (OJ). Finally, it was awarded to her in 1991. By then, Mary had retired from UWI but she was still a member of the council. Her contributions were missed on the council because of the guidance that she gave to members and the chair whenever she thought that it was needed. In a reflective mood, Theresa Boyne concluded, "We miss her on council. We do miss her contribution, as we could always count on Dr Seivwright. Whatever she takes on to do, we know that she is going to do it. And she is going to do it well. We could always count on her for that." Health reasons, and in particular, failing eyesight, and the desire to write a book on the history of nursing in the Caribbean impelled her to resign from the Nursing Council.

Caribbean Activist

While it would appear that the focus to here has been dominated by Mary's contributions to Jamaica, this would be misleading, as students at UWI came from many of the Caribbean islands. Her impact on them was the same as it was for those within her island home, and her influence in promoting the profession was felt beyond Jamaica.

Mary maintained her active interest and association with events in the Caribbean in nursing throughout her career, regardless of her physical location. Distance did not hinder her attendance at meetings and conferences. It was also a fortunate coincidence that her advisory role in the ICN facilitated her travels to the region and its environs. A central source for her input was the CNO, which held its meeting every two years in different islands. One of her earliest addresses was at the sixth biennial conference of the CNO held in 1968 at Mary Seacole House in Kingston. At that time, Mary was the chief project nurse with the Comprehensive Child Care Project at the Albert Einstein College of Medicine/Montefiore Hospital in New York. The theme of the conference was "The Role of the Nurse in the Changing Caribbean". Her comments are worthy of noting here.

> It would appear . . . that the most eminent occupants of various social roles – those who have been immortalized for their contributions – are they who were able to add other dimensions to their perception of the social situation. They possessed the capacity to project themselves into the future and to sense the demands and expectations of a generation yet unborn . . . they possessed the courage not only to articulate these perceptions but to take positive action to implement them. In other words, if you would be a worthy role-bearer, irrespective of your status, you cannot, you must not be content merely to gear your performance to the situation *as is* but to what, in your best judgment, the situation *should be*. You cannot, you must not be satisfied with merely the 'status quo', regardless of how peaceful and comfortable this posture promises to become. Instead, you must be willing and ready to act as agents of progressive change, and count it a privilege to participate in the turbulence and hardship that usually accompany such human events [emphasis mine].[22]

Without a doubt, Mary lived up to those words she so ardently delivered to her colleagues. There was never any discrepancy between Mary's words and her actions.

The ANEU played a part in the formation of the Regional Nursing Body and linkages were also forged with the Faculty of Education, UWI. When Mary was on this body, she would have come into contact again with Nita Barrow, at that time the PAHO/WHO nursing advisor, heading the regional project on evaluation of schools of nursing. Both of them would be in different roles now, no longer teacher and pupil but colleagues on a similar mission: to improve standards of nursing education and patient care in the Caribbean. By virtue of her role as director of the ANEU, UWI, Mary was a member of the newly formed regional body. At the inaugural meeting of the Regional Nursing Body in December 1972, in Georgetown, Guyana, the first business of the meeting was the election of the officers. Voting by secret ballot for the executive of the body, the members unanimously elected were Dr Mary Seivwright; Ena Walters, matron of the Queen Elizabeth Hospital, Barbados, as chairman of the body; and Hilda Bowen, principal nursing officer of the Bahamas. The Regional Nursing Body met annually, with each country in turn hosting the meeting. The executive and subcommittees met in the interim as often as was necessary to complete projects and assigned tasks.[23]

Mary's involvement with nursing education in the Caribbean became even more intensive than in the past because of her role as director of the ANEU. Her knowledge and expertise in educational matters were effectively utilized as there was a need to revise the curriculum in the schools of nursing in the Caribbean, and to set standards for those schools. This need had emanated from the results of the survey of the schools in 1966. Her involvement included the development of criteria for the evaluation of the schools of nursing in the Caribbean as well as a member of the three-person regional team which went to Guyana. She also participated in the development of the regional nursing examinations which were intended to facilitate reciprocity between the islands.

At interisland conferences, Mary was an outspoken critic on nursing matters, especially if she felt that inadequate consideration was being given to the consequences of taking a particular action. Such a critical approach did not always sit well with many of her nursing colleagues. However, there were those who found her criticisms valid: "I would rather it that way, it was all for the good because she would give a critical view of an opinion where people would not say anything. But I found that was a blessing in many instances because in the end it would turn out that she was correct in what she was proposing."[24] This was the viewpoint of Valerie Foster, retired principal nursing officer and former director of schools of nursing in Trinidad and Tobago. She viewed Mary as an advocate for nursing who helped to direct the course of events, not only in Jamaica but for the Caribbean. Beulah Duke, a nurse educator from Trinidad confirmed that Mary was a powerful and assertive speaker: "For us in these parts she was the first 'doctor' nurse... Very confident of herself. Knows about nursing from the grassroots level to the highest level. Cannot be defied by anyone."[25]

These women also shared another side of Mary, which was observed at official social events where she was most warm, very open and friendly. Beulah, who by chance was Mary's roommate at the CNO conference in Bermuda, said, "She is a very warm person. Very concerned about individuals. She knew the students by name and their personal problems... so she would remember those things... In other words, what she was, what she seemed to be academically, on the personal level she's not." A similar view of her warmth and concern for others was narrated by Enid Lawrence who worked with Mary in a number of different roles and in the three organizations the ANEU, the NAJ, and the Nursing Council, and got to know her well.

Mary the Senator

When were the seeds laid for Mary's political involvement? It is hard to say as Mary was always an activist. Caribbean women, by and large, play a subservient role to men, particularly in economic and social areas. A double standard of sexuality exists and women are frequently forced to hide their potential talents and abilities.[26] Mary had no intention of conforming to the prescribed role for women. As a young girl growing up, she was determined to move out of her rural home and not become trapped into marriage and multiple pregnancies. Mary was seen by many as aggressive. It took courage to surmount the barriers of race, colour and social class. It could be argued that it was her so-called aggressive behaviour that got her what she wanted. She fought for her beliefs and for her rights and for those of nurses, and by extension of all women, since the vast majority of nurses still are women. Her approach intimidated men, including physicians and politicians, and many of her own sex.

Her broad concern for her country can be demonstrated by a few examples, such as her address to the nineteenth annual summer school in August 1967, which suggested a beginning to her later political involvement. Among other things, she urged nurses to become involved in the affairs of their island nation through participation in the war against illiteracy, poverty, crime, disease, and the many social ills that affected the country. A few years later she gave a clarion call to Jamaican nurses to promote the cause, not only of nursing but of the country as a whole, as she pleaded with them to become not only participants in their professional organization but also in the affairs of their young nation as well. Again, in May 1972, when she opened the Nurses' Week celebrations, Mary spoke on the participation of nurses in policy making. It was the theme of the International Council of Nurses for that year but, as usual, it was her philosophical perspective linked to events and issues in Jamaica that always informed her choices. She encouraged her audience to participate in the development of their country:

For the first time in the history of this country, *public participation in the administration of national affairs* has been declared a policy of the Government. This, I believe, is welcome news to all citizens. As Jamaican nurses, however, the declaration should be of particular significance to us, since for a long time we have been concerned about various aspects of participation . . . some organized efforts are being made by nurses in several parts of the island to involve themselves in community projects of one sort or another . . . You need to keep abreast of developments in nursing education and practice and be aware of changes in the science and technology of medicine and health, in developed as well as developing countries. *You must be knowledgeable about and sensitive to socioeconomic and cultural conditions in your country and in the region* ... Let us resolve to give, in fullest measure, our whole hearted support and cooperation in all those activities which go to build a viable, just, and healthy nation [emphasis mine].[27]

When Mary returned to Jamaica for good in the 1970s, she saw the rise of the women's liberation movement and the global concern for the role of women in the world – the struggle for equality. The United Nations proclaimed 1975 International Women's Year, in order to focus attention on the poverty and plight of women especially in the developing world. Mary was invited to give the address at the first annual meeting of the St Matthew's "Adventurers", an Anglican church group. She examined some of the common myths regarding the role of women, and provided challenges for her audience for the future. Her words are instructive as they exemplify the congruency between her thought and actions. She expressed some of her thoughts this way: "The day cannot be far off when the women of the world should be able to attain full development of their potentialities, complete self-actualization, and their maximum contribution as citizens, unfettered by the stultifying myths by which we have lived."[28]

On the international scene, about this time, Mary was elected to the board of directors of the ICN where formerly she had worked as an advisor. This was a signal honour, as these positions are highly competitive and political with intense lobbying by member organizations to get their candidate elected. Mary was a first once more as the first West Indian to be elected to the board of the ICN. During her tenure, Mary chaired the subcommittee on membership of the board. The role of this committee was to consider applications for membership in the ICN by member associations. Among the countries admitted was St Lucia. This association was visited by Mary when she was advisor to the ICN and Jamaica was the sponsor for St Lucia's admittance to the ICN conference held in Japan in 1977.

All these activities laid the groundwork for her more formal political involvement in Jamaica in the 1980s. Mary was a true feminist, whether or not she or others labelled her as such. She looked at the world in which she lived and worked and developed strategies and approaches to confront the system and to enhance her self-esteem and that of nurses, and at the same time promoted their value to their society. Her approach is consistent with classic liberal feminist thinking, where nurses are exhorted to become leaders and managers of change within the patriarchal workplace and system.[29]

By 1980 Mary was president once more of the NAJ. Even more important was her swearing in as a member of the Senate, selected by the People's National Party, in December 1980. This honour – the first nurse ever to sit in the Senate – was

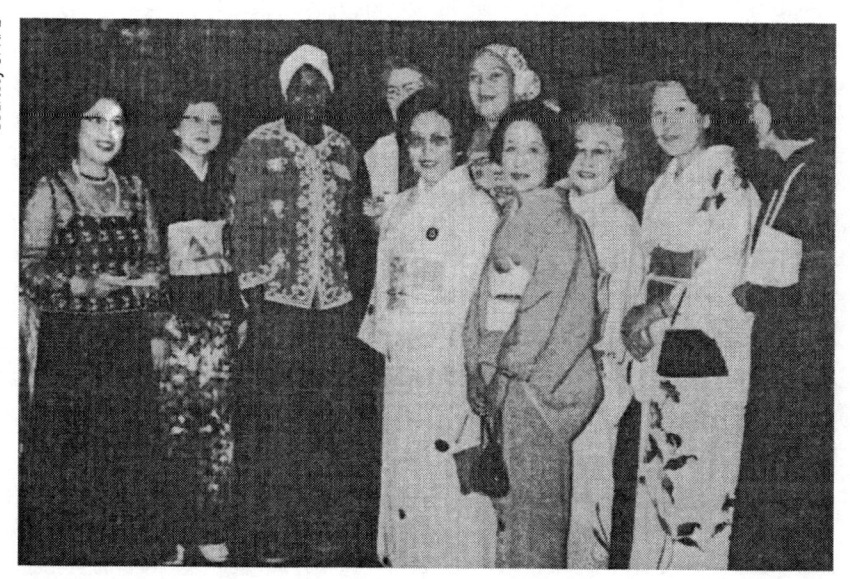

Mary (third from left) at a reception with the Japanese Nursing Association, fourteenth quadrennial congress, International Council of Nurses, Tokyo, Japan, 1977

highlighted in the *Gleaner*. She was soon appointed to the Committee of Privileges. Mary participated actively on the Rent Assessment and Control Bill when she spoke eloquently on the deficiencies and inconsistencies in the content of the bill.

In November 1981, during her term on the Senate, Mary was the victim of a vicious attack by unknown assailants as she entered her home. The injuries she sustained necessitated a stay in hospital. The condolences of Senate as well as the violence in the country were recorded by the president of the Senate. On her return to the Senate, her zeal and enthusiasm never abated. She served her country in the Senate until 1984 when her term expired.[30]

It was fitting that Mary would eventually receive recognition for her contributions to the status and role of Jamaican women. In 1987, on International Women's Day, the Bureau of Women's Affairs bestowed on her the Woman of Distinction award.

Mary retired from her position as director of the ANEU at UWI in the following year. She had intended to write a book on Caribbean nursing and to enjoy her gardening, which is a lifelong passion. Unfortunately, ill health, particularly failing eyesight, has limited her activity in both these areas. Nevertheless, Mary's presence and input into nursing affairs, orally and in the written word, continued unabated. As late as 1991, three years after her retirement, Mary pleaded with her readers, nurses, to undertake research, as it was the imperative of the era in which they lived. She reminded those who had research talents to invest them in the scientific study of their practice regardless of how small the returns might be, for "the critically important thing is that you made use of your gift".[31] And, undoubtedly, Mary used her gift.

The 1990s were to herald further accolades. In 1991 the Government of Jamaica honoured her as the first Jamaican nurse to be awarded the Order of Jamaica. She became the Honourable Dr Mary Jane Seivwright. In May 1992 she received an honorary degree, Doctor of Humanities, from Capital University, Columbus, Ohio. In her citation, the nominator said:

Capital University nursing students took clinical as well as classroom courses in Jamaica, an opportunity rarely afforded to nursing students in this country. The bestowing of this Honorary Degree on Dr Mary Jane Seivwright, a nurse highly esteemed in Jamaica and well-respected in international circles, is a fitting expression of our deep appreciation to all of the nurses and educators of Jamaica. In honouring Dr Seivwright, we would be honouring all the students and nurses in the global community whom she has influenced. This Honorary degree would be an apt tribute for this remarkable woman.[32]

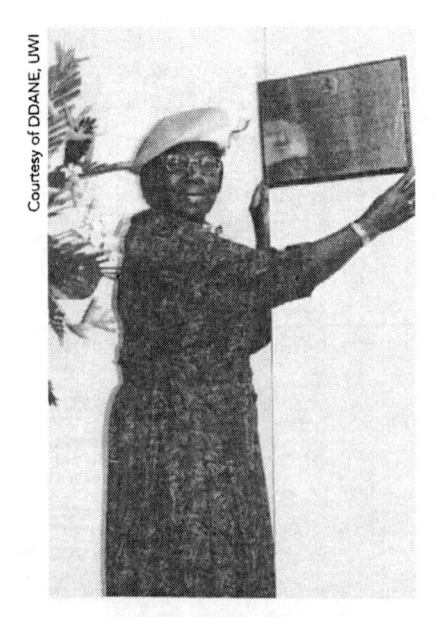

Mary, at the naming ceremony of the Mary Jane Seivwright Building, UWI, Mona, Jamaica, 4 April 1997

The final accolade for Mary, at the time of writing, came in April 1997 when at the Department of Advanced Nursing Education, on the grounds of UWI, a plaque was unveiled naming the building the Mary Jane Seivwright Building. It is said that the building on the campus grounds was the result of Mary's almost single-handed efforts. It was a well-deserved tribute to a woman who devoted her life to the advancement of nursing.

Today, Mary still lives alone high up in Stony Hill in her beloved "Croton

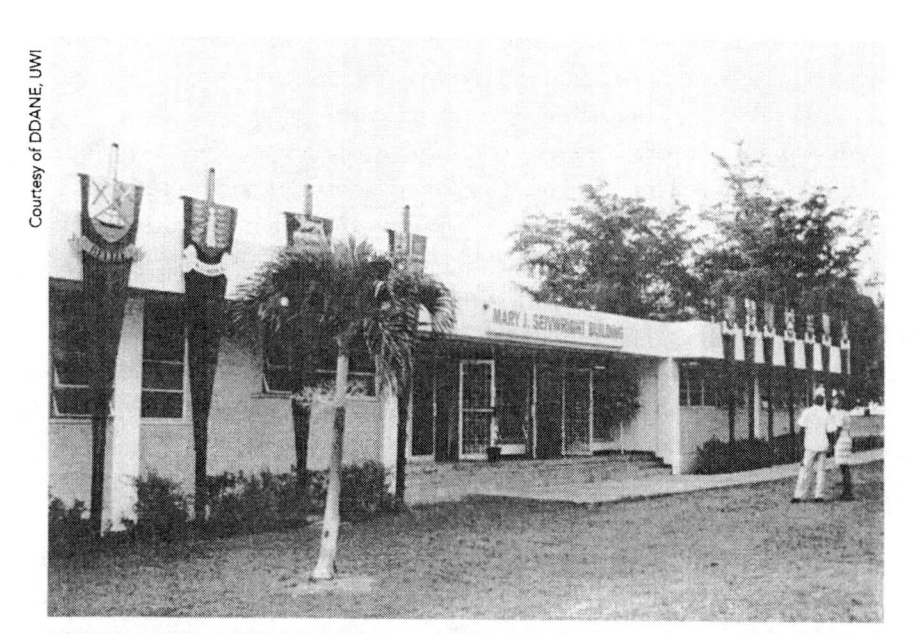

The Mary Jane Seivwright Building draped with the CARICOM countries' coats of arms and pennants representing the countries of all students who came to the Department of Advanced Nursing Education during Mary's tenure at UWI, 1997

Villa", so named because of the profusion of exotic and varied colourful crotons (which she planted) that line the walkway to her home. Relatively far from Kingston, her choice of location was deliberate. The setting is spectacular, commanding a view of the sea and the mountains. During Mary's formative years, there was a striking correlation between race, income and residential location. At that time, the residential sections of the suburbs rose gradually toward the Blue Mountains and the racial complexion of the residents changed and the income rose appreciably with the elevation. The whites and the wealthy coloureds lived above the 500-feet level, while the black workers, who constituted the great majority of the population, lived in the congested slums of the lowlands.[33] Where Mary lives now is a visible sign of the changed times and her social status, although it could be argued that since her birthplace was in the Dry Harbour Mountains of St Ann, she would choose to live in the hills. The land is lush with fruit, shrubs, flowers and abundant vegetables which Mary plants and tends herself. As Merel Hanson said, "She would not leave that house, even at this stage, because she loves to be in the soil, work with her hands . . . and offer you something out of her garden." Her intense love of the land and its fruits is central to her being, as is her spirituality. Those two dimensions are undoubtedly what sustain Mary and replenish her energies to continue to give of herself so seemingly endlessly.

Father Robert Thompson of St Andrew's Parish in Half Way Tree, Kingston, was Mary's pastor for over a decade when he was rector of St Jude's Church in Stony Hill. He portrayed her as a tower of strength physically, spiritually and intellectually. Her involvement in the life of the church was exemplary. She was a member of the church council and represented the church on many occasions. He gave his view of her deep faith: "She is a deeply religious woman. Knows her Bible very well, reads her Bible regularly and literally feeds on God's words for her life. And that has sustained her, no doubt, over the years and more or less gave her the foundation and the base to serve. And it serves her well. A community person. Mary loves people. And I remember from time to time we would have members in the congregation who need care, who need attention, who need to be cared for in ways that many people don't get involved in because it demands so much of your time. And she would care for these people, get their groceries, go visit them. If there were wounds to be mended she would do that . . . the wounds were not only physical. Social and emotional needs she would deal with. So, from the point of view from her own Christian life, it was not just one of solitary reflection of the word, it was lived out in her service within the community."[34]

Father Thompson and his family often visit Mary and he, like others, has shared his concern for her safety and well-being, living so far away and on her own. A robbery on her premises in 1996, when her china and silver cutlery were stolen, left her feeling very vulnerable, but she was adamant that she would not move from her house. Father Thompson expressed sadness that in the evening of her years she was alone and so far away and disappointed that he, and many others, could not persuade her to do otherwise. Yet he appeared comforted that he was able to provide her with support in times when she needed it.

Mary's isolation and her failing eyesight have remained a source of concern to her colleagues who, while they telephone her regularly, visit less frequently because of the distance. "Croton Villa" is Mary's pride and joy. It epitomizes her struggle to climb upwards in a symbolic and real sense as she rose from a less privileged position in life and had to fight against all odds to break the barriers and to reach the top, where she is today.

It would be appropriate to close with Mary's own words from her stimulating and scholarly address to the summer school of the NAJ more than thirty years ago. She exhorted others to do what she in fact has done all her life:

You must identify yourself with your community – in this case, our island nation. You cannot afford to be 'in it' yet not 'of it'. The problems of the nation must become your personal concern; its progress toward mature and responsible statehood, your personal objective. You must feel that you have a personal stake in its future, because you are an important part of it . . . with active and meaningful participation in community affairs. I look forward to the day when . . . we will be prominent among those who labour ceaselessly in the cause of social progress, moral decency and responsible nationhood.[35]

Mary Jane Seivwright, born poor, black and bright, blazed her way to the top of her profession and her society. An ardent advocate for nurses and nursing, she is an incandescent light leading the way. It is up to others to follow.

NOTES

1. Marina Andrewin Staine, personal interview, June 1996. All material quoted from Staine is from this interview.
2. Thelma Campbell, personal interview, June 1996. All material quoted from Campbell is from this interview.
3. M.J. Seivwright, "Report of the Advanced Nursing Education Unit: Historical Highlights and Present Considerations" (Mona, Jamaica: Department of Social and Preventive Medicine, UWI, 1977); "A Proposal for a Bachelor of Science Degree in Nursing" (Department of Social and Preventive Medicine, UWI, January 1970), 13.
4. *Daily Gleaner*, 5 August 1974.
5. Seivwright, "Report of the Advanced Nursing Education Unit", 1–4.
6. Memorandum and attachments from Mary J. Seivwright to Aston Preston.
7. Sir Kenneth Standard, personal interview, June 1996. All material quoted from Sir Kenneth Standard is from this interview.
8. Mary Grant, personal interview, June 1996. All material quoted from Grant is from this interview.
9. Seivwright, "Report of the Advanced Nursing Education Unit", 28–39.
10. *Nursing in Jamaica: Blueprint for Progress* (Kingston, Jamaica: Nurses' Association of Jamaica, 1972), 22.
11. Project HOPE (Health Opportunities for People Everywhere) was established by Dr William Walsh of Bethesda, Maryland, in the 1950s. Its mission is to help to improve health care around the world, in the less developed areas, by educating health professionals. The essence of Project HOPE is teaching through partnership. All of the

people of HOPE work in various capacities to help people help themselves. Its international headquarters are located in Millwood, Virginia.

12. M.J. Seivwright, "The Nurse Practitioner Programme (NPP) in Jamaica" (address given at the first graduation ceremony of the Nurse Practitioner Programme, Faculty of Medicine, UWI, 28 June 1978). See also minutes of the meeting of the Committee on Nursing Education, 21 December 1977, UWI (File ref. C104/2–53, 30 May 1978).
13. This protocol manual is well established and now serves everyone in all clinics. It has become a standard of practice.
14. Yvonne Young Reid, personal interview, June 1996. All material quoted from Reid is from this interview.
15. Hermi Hewitt, personal interview, June 1996. All material quoted from Hewitt is from this interview.
16. Pearlie Esteen, personal interview, June 1996. All material quoted from Esteen is from this interview.
17. Merel Hanson, personal interview, June 1996. Unless otherwise indicated, material quoted from Hanson is from this interview.
18. *Nursing in Jamaica*, 1–26.
19. G. Lewis, *The Growth of the Modern West Indies* (New York: Monthly Review Press, 1968), 193. See also A. Bakan, *Ideology and Class Conflict in Jamaica* (Montreal: McGill-Queen's University Press, 1990), 135–40, for a full exposition of the political and economic situation in Jamaica; as well as P. Hay Ho Sang, "The Development of Nursing Education in Jamaica, West Indies: 1900–1975" (DEd diss., Teachers' College, Columbia University, 1984), 235–37; and M.J. Seivwright, "Socio-Economic Welfare of Jamaican Nurses: Highlights of NAJ Accomplishments", *Jamaican Nurse* 21 (1981): 21–23, regarding the economic conditions of nurses.
20. M. Hanson, citation to the Hon Dr Mary Jane Seivwright on the occasion of naming the boardroom of the NAJ, Kingston, Jamaica, in her honor, 8 May 1995.
21. Theresa Boyne, personal interview, June 1996. All material quoted from Boyne is from this interview.
22. M.J. Seivwright, "The Nature of Role", *Jamaican Nurse* 25 (1986): 12–14.
23. E.K. Walters, *Nursing: A History from the Late Eighteenth–Late Twentieth Century Barbados* (Bridgetown, Barbados: E.K. Walters, 1995), 97–105.
24. Valerie Foster, personal interview, April 1996. All material quoted from Foster is from this interview.
25. Beulah Duke, personal interview, April 1996. All material quoted from Duke is from this interview.
26. F. Henry and P. Wilson, "The Status of Women in Caribbean Societies: An Overview of Their Social, Economic, and Sexual Roles", *Social and Economic Studies* 24 (1975): 165–98.

27. M.J. Seivwright, "The Nurses' Participation in Policy-Making", *Jamaican Nurse* 12 (1972): 12–14.
28. M.J. Seivwright, "Organization for Effective Participation", *Jamaican Nurse* 11 (1971): 5.
29. M. Kramer and C. Schmalenberg, "Magnet Hospitals: Institutions of Excellence", Part 1, *Journal of Nursing Administration* 18, no. 1 (1988): 13–24.
30. *Debates*. Session 1981–1982, 27 November 1981 (Kingston, Jamaica: Government Printing Office, 1981).
31. M.J. Seivwright, guest editorial, *Jamaican Nurse* 29 (1991): 3.
32. L. Talabere, e-mail message to the author, 5 September 1997.
33. P. Blanshard, *Democracy and Empire in the Caribbean* (New York: Macmillan), 86–87.
34. Father Robert Thompson, personal interview, June 1996. All material quoted from Thompson is from this interview.
35. M.J. Seivwright, "You, Your Profession and the Community", *Jamaican Nurse* 7 (1967): 31.

Conclusion

West Indian society has been shaped by the historical forces of colonization, slavery, sugar production, the plantation system and emancipation. For these English-speaking islands, the avenue of communication during colonial days was between the individual islands and London rather than between the territories themselves. This led to a sense of separate identity within each island, while at the same time the massive forces at play over the entire area left a common historical experience and a common imprint upon the people.[1]

During the colonial era, when Nita, Ben and Mary were born, Caribbean women were a silent neglected group. Improvements and reforms rarely touched their lives. Yet they played a major role in the economic life of the region. They worked in a variety of roles as domestic workers, sales clerks, professional workers, such as nurses and teachers, and government clerks. Professional women made a major contribution to the society at great personal sacrifice and were expected to be steeped in European culture. They tutored children, taught Sunday school, and acted as consultants in family and community affairs. In addition, they carried out the nurturing role of women – they loved, inspired, motivated, and helped children of the poor to achieve goals that, for them, were unattainable.[2]

It is not surprising that Nita and Ben entered nursing, as there were few options open to them. They were born of middle-class professional parents and were deeply influenced by them. Nita's father, a pastor, and her uncle, a physician, were activists who championed the cause of the poor and the underprivileged, so she grew up within a family circle that was socially aware and committed. She, like them, would become involved in religious, health and social organizations as an activist for the causes of nurses and women.

Ben's mother was very involved in community endeavours and her father, a pharmacist, in both church and community work. Another major role model for Ben during her teens was one of the earliest black professional women, a social worker, who was an advocate for poor women and children. Ben admired her and became involved in community activities for the elderly and the poor during her high school years. Although she married shortly after graduating as a nurse, Ben's husband, a physician, was most supportive of her career and multiple voluntary endeavours.

Mary, unlike the other two, was born of parents with very modest means. She looked at the society and conditions in which she found herself and was determined to rise above them. With an innate drive and the help of an Anglican minister during her tender years, she sought the route of teaching prior to her entry into nursing.

A central element in these women's lives was the prevailing political and social climate of the 1930s. The deteriorating social and economic conditions in the islands led to widespread social and political unrest, and there was much disaffection in the society. Nursing was predominantly an apprenticeship system with British sisters and matrons occupying the leadership positions in the health services. Nita and Ben both had the vision to realize that nurses needed to unify if standards of education and practice were to be improved. By 1946 Nita became the catalyst in organizing Jamaican nurses into an association. At the same time, Ben spearheaded the movement to unite nurses from the north and south of Trinidad into one association. Each served as president of their local nurses' association from 1946 to 1948, frequently communicating with each other since both organizations were attempting to achieve registration for nurses. Registration for nurses was achieved in Trinidad by 1950 and by 1951 in Jamaica. It was a major accomplishment because it meant reciprocity with Great Britain, held up as the gold standard. The year 1953 saw both Jamaica and Trinidad gaining membership in the ICN at the conference in Brazil. Nita's work undoubtedly had an impact on Mary who was then a nursing student. She was impressed by the importance of the movement and the appearance of black nursing leaders working to advance the interests of Jamaican nurses. A few decades later, she herself took up the mantle at the NAJ as president and made nursing a force to be reckoned with throughout her many years with the association and the Nursing Council. These three women worked to prepare nurses for leadership, each in her own way, whether through facilitating nurses to get scholarships to study abroad or getting postdiploma courses organized locally, or administering and teaching university courses.

Another similarity was their dedication to the field of public health. Long before WHO advocated the concept of primary health care in 1978, Nita, Ben and Mary each had a vision of nursing that went beyond the narrow confines of caring for the sick and reached out to the broader realm of health care. They all gained advanced preparation in the field of public health as they recognized that health care entailed preventive measures and also the education of women in all dimensions. Nita studied public health at the University of Toronto, Ben at the Royal Sanitary Institute in London, and Mary at the West Indies School of Public Health, UWI, where Nita was then a tutor. Nita's community work with the International Council of Adult Education was extensive and with the CMC where her major focus was primary health care and the role of women. Ben's focus in public health was in the voluntary sector, as a founder of the Chest and Heart Association, where her activities centred on rehabilitation, counselling and assisting clients to attend clinics. Mary worked as a public health nurse for many years in a rural community in Jamaica, serving the poor and the disadvantaged. Her continuing concern for community health was also seen in her introduction and development of the Nurse Practitioner Programme when she became the first director of the ANEU at the UWI.

In the 1940s and 1950s, the prevailing political climate was the movement for unification of the islands. Consequently, there was a convergence of these three women, propelled by events in the region. During those years, several regional developments became unifying initiatives, including the establishment of the UCWI, which enabled scholars to study in the Caribbean; the first medical school to prepare West Indian physicians, the UCHWI; the CNO; a regional survey of schools of nursing; and the Regional Nursing Body.

Nita, Ben and Mary each played significant roles in those initiatives and have left their mark on nursing education and nursing service to the present time. Nita was the first West Indian nurse to be matron of the UCHWI. In 1959, at the historic conference of Caribbean nursing administrators which met in Barbados, she, as principal nursing officer of Jamaica, was the secretary to that conference which led to the formation of the Regional Nursing Body. Ben and Mary were at the conference, Ben representing the Nursing Council of Trinidad and Tobago, and Mary as a delegate. This was just the beginning of their mutual influence, as their paths would continually cross. Ben was frequently an advisor on constitutional matters for the CNO and Mary was an active delegate and keynote speaker for that organization.

Their greater collective impact came in the 1960s with the regional survey of schools of nursing. Nita was the first Caribbean regional project director for the survey; Ben served on the steering committee and later the advisory committee to that project, which then became a board of review for the evaluation of the schools of nursing in the thirteen territories; and Mary was a major contributor to and player in that project. Later, the Commonwealth Nursing Seminar, a precursor of the Regional Nursing Body formed in 1972, provided the venue for them to use their influence collectively for the improvement of nursing education in the region. Nita was a resource person in her role as a PAHO/WHO Caribbean nursing advisor, and Mary, an advisor with the ICN, was a member of the budget committee for the conference. Mary, the first local director of the ANEU, later became an elected executive officer of the body. The paths of these three women intersected at a critical period in the history of nursing in the region. It was a transitional stage for the Caribbean as a whole, and for nursing specifically, as indigenous nurses worked rigorously to wrest the leadership mantle from the British in nursing service and education. Nita, Ben and Mary, among others, were in the forefront of that struggle, not merely assuming leadership positions but, rather, ensuring through example that standards of excellence were attained and maintained in education and practice.

All three of them made an international impact. Nita became president of the World YWCA, director of the CMC of the WCC, ambassador to the United Nations and, ultimately, governor general of her home island, Barbados. Ben was a national representative and a board member of the ICN, an ardent island representative for the League of Women Voters (the British Commonwealth League), the International Alliance of Women, the Soroptimists, and other international voluntary agencies at meetings internationally. Mary held the post of nursing research project director at Teachers' College, Columbia University, chief project nurse at the Montefiore Hospital and Medical Center in New York City, and international nursing advisor with the ICN. Thus they all played an active role in the development, education, and well-being of women through political and social action locally, regionally and beyond.

Nursing today in the English-speaking Caribbean is an organized profession, with professional associations and nursing councils to ensure that standards for education and practice are met. It has gained recognition internationally through membership in the ICN, and its present nursing leaders in education and the health services are well-educated and indigenous to the Caribbean. Those who benefited from their examples can be found in a variety of leadership roles as hospital chief executive officers, matrons, directors of nursing service and education, instructors, clinical specialists at home and abroad, and nurse practitioners. It is largely due to the vision and dedication of these nursing pioneers that nursing education in the Caribbean has a sound curriculum. Those who followed in their steps continue to seek improvements for education and practice of nurses. Associate, certificate and university degree programmes have been introduced to meet the health and social needs of the society as it changes.

Nita, Ben and Mary have left their stamp of zeal, enthusiasm, courage, persistence and dedication to high standards to future generations. Each one was unique. Dame Nita was unassuming and unpretentious, and always made others feel special; Ben was forthright, a storehouse of knowledge and information, and highly principled; Mary was impressive, formidable and brilliant. Sticklers for detail, with a remarkable capacity to recall minutiae, they were the undisputed leaders and role models for nurses and women of the region. What served as the fundamental core of their passion and caring? It is undeniably their deep spirituality. Their profound and abiding faith in God enabled them to persist where others might have given up. They expressed their deep faith in service to others through the modality of caring. All three were seeking much the same goal – to be of service to all, but to women and nurses in particular. Again they differed in the manifestation of this faith. Dame Nita became director of the CMC of the WCC; Ben and Dr Mary were actively involved with their particular churches, Roman Catholic and Anglican. Apart from this accepted route through the established church, their concern for the status of women nationally and, in Dame Nita's case, internationally, saw them addressing the needs of the less privileged through their active participation in educational, social and health activities for women. I think they would agree that these qualities were gifts from God. Gifts that they shared with humanity.

Nursing has been deemed a woman's occupation, and, like the history of black women, has suffered in the neglect of its recorded history. Nursing in the Caribbean has many hidden heroines. I chose to open the window on only three such women. Their striking similarities were their passion for nursing and their care for the well-being of women, their unswerving pursuit of excellence, the articulate expression of their beliefs and the translation of those beliefs into practice for nursing, health care and the welfare of women. Whatever mission they undertook, they did it tenaciously and with a fervour and vigour parallelled by few. Individually and collectively they propelled Caribbean nursing to the forefront politically. This is the legacy of these three women.

NOTE

1. G. Lewis, *The Growth of the Modern West Indies* (New York: Monthly Review Press, 1968).
2. T. Thompson, "Caribbean Womanhood: A Past Denied, a Future Promised", in *The Caribbean Issues of Emergence: Socioeconomic and Political Perspectives*, ed. Vincent MacDonald (Washingon, DC: University Press of America, 1980), 200–201.

Bibliography

Abrahams, P. *Jamaica: An Island Mosaic.* London: HMSO, 1958.

Ayearst, M. *The British West Indies.* New York: New York University Press, 1960.

Bakan, A. *Ideology and Class Conflict in Jamaica.* Montreal: McGill-Queen's University Press, 1990.

Barnard, Celine. "Dame Nita Barrow: An Outstanding Woman". *Bajan,* January/February 1986.

Barrow, R. Nita. "Nursing: The Art, Science and Vocation in Evolution". *Contact* 59 (December 1980).

Barrow, R. Nita. "The Role of Women in International Development". Address given at the University of Alberta, Edmonton, Alberta, 10 March 1987.

Barrow, R. Nita. "Nursing: A New Tomorrow". *International Nursing Review* 36, no. 5 (1989).

Beckles, H. *A History of Barbados: From Amerindian Settlement to Nation-State.* Cambridge: Cambridge University Press, 1990.

Blackman, F.W. *Dame Nita: Caribbean Woman, World Citizen.* Kingston, Jamaica: Ian Randle Publishers, 1995.

Blanshard, P. *Democracy and Empire in the Caribbean.* New York: Macmillan, 1947.

Brathwaite, L. "Social Stratification in Trinidad". *Social and Economic Studies* 2 (1953).

Brereton, B. *A History of Modern Trinidad 1783–1962.* London: Heinemann, 1981.

Bryce-Boodoo, M. "A Fresh Look at Nursing Education in Trinidad and Tobago". In *The Nursing Council of Trinidad and Tobago Twenty-fifth Anniversary 1950–1975.* Port of Spain, Trinidad: Key Publications, 1975.

Bibliography

Carnegie, M.E. *The Path We Tread: Blacks in Nursing Worldwide 1854–1994*, 3d ed. New York: National League for Nursing Press, 1995.

Carpenter, H.M. "The University of Toronto School of Nursing: Agent of Change". In *Nursing in a Changing Society*, edited by Mary Innis. Toronto: University of Toronto Press, 1970.

Christian Medical Commission/World Council of Churches. "Health Care for All: A New Priority". *Contact* 26 (April 1975).

Christian Medical Commission/World Council of Churches. "The Annual Meeting of the Christian Medical Commission". *Contact* 39 (April 1977).

Christian Medical Commission/World Council of Churches. "CMC Study/Enquiry: The Roots". *Contact* 51 (June 1979).

Clarke, C. "Society and Electoral Politics in Trinidad and Tobago". In *Society and Politics*, edited by C. Clarke. New York: St Martin's Press, 1991.

Cochrane, N., et al. *J.R. Kidd: An International Legacy of Learning*. Vancouver: Centre for Continuing Education, University of British Columbia, 1986.

Comissiong, L.M. "Health Services in the British Caribbean: 1935–1969". *Caribbean Medical Journal* 30 (1970).

Covey, S.R. *The Seven Habits of Highly Effective People*. New York: Simon and Schuster, 1990.

Davis, A.T. *Early Black American Leaders in Nursing: Architects for Integration and Equity*. Sudbury, Mass.: Jones and Bartlett, 1999.

De Verteuil, E. "The Urgent Need for a Medical and Health Policy for Trinidad". *Caribbean Medical Journal* 5, no. 3 (1943).

Dolly, B. "The Development of Nursing Education in Trinidad and Tobago". Typescript, 1966.

Durdin, J. *They Became Nurses: A History of Nursing in South Australia, 1830–1980*. North Sydney: Allen and Unwin, 1991.

Federal Government of the West Indies, Barbados. Report of Conference of Nursing Administrators, Bridgetown, Barbados, 31 August–6 September 1959.

Gardner, J.W. *Excellence: Can We Be Equal and Excellent Too?* New York: Harper and Row, 1962.

Gibran, K. *The Prophet*. New York: Knopf, 1961.

Grayson, J.H.F. "The Nurses' Association of Trinidad and Tobago". DEd diss., Teachers' College, Columbia University, 1989.

Hansen, M. Citation to the Hon Dr Mary Jane Seivwright on the occasion of naming the boardroom of the NAJ, Kingston, Jamaica, in her honour, 8 May 1995.

Hay Ho Sang, P. "The Development of Nursing Education in Jamaica, West Indies: 1900–1975". DEd diss., Teachers' College, Columbia University, 1984.

Bibliography

Henry, F., and P. Wilson. "The Status of Women in Caribbean Societies: An Overview of Their Social, Economic and Sexual Roles". *Social and Economic Studies* 24 (1975).

Hezekiah, J. "The Development of Nursing Education in Trinidad and Tobago: 1956–1986". PhD diss., University of Alberta, Edmonton, 1987.

Hezekiah, J. "Nursing Leadership and the Colonial Heritage". *Image: Journal of Nursing Scholarship* 20, no. 3 (1988).

Hezekiah, J. "The Development of Health Care Policies in Trinidad and Tobago: Autonomy or Domination?" *International Journal of Health Services* 19, no. 1 (1989).

Hezekiah, J. "Post-colonial Nursing Education in Trinidad and Tobago". *Advances in Nursing Science* 12, no. 2 (1990).

Hine, D.C. *Black Women in White: Racial Conflict and Cooperation in the Nursing Profession, 1890–1950*. Bloomington: Indiana University Press, 1989.

Hunte, G. *Jamaica*. London: B.T. Batsford, 1976.

Jamaica. Parliament. *Debates* (Session 1981–1982, 27 November 1981). Kingston, Jamaica: Government Printing Office, 1981.

Kidd, R. *Whilst Time is Burning: A Report on Education for Development*. Ottawa: International Development Research Centre, 1974.

Khanna, S.K. *History of Nursing in India from 1947–1989*. Missouri: Cape Girardeau, 1991.

Kodamer, K. *Nursing in Japan*. Tokyo: Nippon Kango Kyokai, Showersznner, 1977.

Kramer, M., and C. Schmalenberg. "Magnet Hospitals: Institutions of Excellence". Parts 1, 2. *Journal of Nursing Administration* 18, nos. 1 and 2 (1988).

Landsberg, M. "World Says Goodbye to One Grand Dame". *Toronto Star*, 23 December 1995.

Laurence, S.M. "The Evolution of the Trinidad Midwife". *Caribbean Medical Journal* 3, no. 4 (1941).

Lewis, G. *The Growth of the Modern West Indies*. New York: Monthly Review Press, 1968.

Lowenthal, D. *West Indian Societies*. London: Oxford University Press, 1972.

Marshall-Burnett, S. "A Brief Reflection on the Life of Mary Seacole 1805–1881". *Jamaican Nurse* 21, no. 2 (1981).

Minister, K. "A Feminist Frame for the Oral History Interview". In *Women's Words: The Feminist Practice of Oral History*, edited by H. Gluck and D. Patai. New York: Routledge, Chapman and Hall, 1991.

Mohammed, P. "Women and Education". In *Women in the Caribbean Project*, vol. 5, edited by Joycelin Massiah. Cave Hill, Barbados: Institute of Social and Economic Research, 1982.

Mussallem, H. *Spotlight on Nursing Education: A Report of the Pilot Project for the Evaluation of Schools of Nursing in Canada*. Ottawa: Canadian Nurses' Association, 1960.

Bibliography

Nurses' Association of Jamaica. *Nursing in Jamaica: Blueprint for Progress*. Kingston, Jamaica: Nurses' Association of Jamaica, 1972.

Pan American Health Organization/World Health Organization. *Survey of Schools of Nursing in the Caribbean Area*. Reports on Nursing no. 6. Washington, DC: PAHO/WHO, 1966.

Pan American Health Organization/World Health Organization. *Resurvey of Schools of Nursing in the Caribbean Area*. Reports on Nursing, no. 15, vol. 1, Nursing Education. Washington, DC: PAHO/WHO, 1971.

Pan American Health Organization/World Health Organization. *WHO Technical Report*, series 633. Washington, DC: PAHO/WHO, 1979.

Reddock, R.E. *Women, Labour and Struggle in Twentieth Century Trinidad and Tobago, 1898–1960*. The Hague: Institute of Social Studies, 1984.

Seivwright, M.J. "You, Your Profession and the Community". *Jamaican Nurse* 7 (1967).

Seivwright, M.J. "A Proposal for a Bachelor of Science Degree in Nursing". Department of Social and Preventive Medicine, UWI Mona, Jamaica. January 1970.

Seivwright, M.J. "Organization for Effective Participation". *Jamaican Nurse* 11 (1971).

Seivwright, M.J. "The Nurses' Participation in Policy-making". *Jamaican Nurse* 12 (1972).

Seivwright, M.J. "The Role of Women: Some Common Myths". *Jamaican Nurse* 15 (1975).

Seivwright, M.J. "Report of the Advanced Nursing Education Unit: Historical Highlights and Present Considerations". Mona, Jamaica: Department of Social and Preventive Medicine, UWI, 1977.

Seivwright, M.J. "The Nurse Practitioner Programme (NPP) in Jamaica". Address given at the first graduation ceremony of the Nurse Practitioner Programme, Faculty of Medicine, UWI, 28 June 1978.

Seivwright, M.J. "Socio-economic Welfare of Jamaican Nurses: Highlights of NAJ Accomplishments". *Jamaican Nurse* 21 (1981).

Seivwright, M.J. "The Florence Nightingale of Jamaica: Mary Seacole". *Jamaican Nurse* 21 (1981).

Seivwright, M.J. "The Nature of Role". *Jamaican Nurse* 25 (1986).

Seivwright, M.J. Guest editorial. *Jamaican Nurse* 29 (1991).

Senior, O. *Working Miracles: Women's Lives in the English-speaking Caribbean*. Cave Hill, Barbados: Institute of Social and Economic Research, 1991.

Splane, R., and V. Splane. *Chief Nursing Officer Positions in National Ministries of Health: Focal Point for Nursing Leadership*. San Francisco: The Regents, School of Nursing, University of California, San Francisco, 1994.

Standard, E. "Dame Nita Barrow". Paper presented at the unveiling of a bust in memory of Dame Nita Barrow, Nurses' Association of Jamaica, Mona, Jamaica, 20 March 1997.

Bibliography

Sunshine, C. *The Caribbean: Survival, Struggle and Sovereignty*. Part I. Ecumenical Program for Interamerican Communication and Action (EPICA). Washington, DC: EPICA, 1973.

Thompson, T. "Caribbean Womanhood: A Past Denied, a Future Promised". In *The Caribbean Issues of Emergence: Socioeconomic and Political Perspectives*, edited by Vincent MacDonald (Washington, DC: University Press of America, 1980).

Thoms, A.B. *Pathfinders: A History of the Progress of Colored Graduate Nurses*. New York: Garland, 1985.

Tree, R. *A History of Barbados*. New York: Random House, 1972.

Trinidad Guardian. Seventy-fifth anniversary edition, 30 August 1992.

Trinidad and Tobago. *Report of the Commission of Enquiry*. M.T. Julien, chairman. Council Paper no. 14. Port of Spain, Trinidad, 1957.

Trinidad and Tobago. Ministry of Health. "Report of First Conference of Caribbean Health Ministers, 11–14 February 1969, Trinidad".

Trinidad and Tobago. Ministry of Health. "Final Report of Second Conference of Caribbean Health Ministers, 28 April–2 May 1970, Barbados".

Trinidad and Tobago Registered Nurses' Association. *Trinidad and Tobago Registered Nurses' Association: Fifty Years of Service, 1930–1980*. Port of Spain, Trinidad: Trinidad and Tobago Registered Nurses' Association, c. 1980.

United Kingdom. Colonial Office. *Report of Commission Trinidad and Tobago Disturbances 1937*. Cmd. 5641, 1938.

United Kingdom. Colonial Office. *Report of the Committee on the Training of Nurses for the Colonies*. Lord Rushcliffe, chairman. Cmd. 6672, 1945.

United Kingdom. Colonial Office. *West India Royal Commission Report*. Cmd. 6607, 1945.

The University of the West Indies. Mona, Jamaica: Public Relations Office, 1994.

Walters, E.K. *Nursing: A History from the Late 18th–Late 20th Century, Barbados*. Bridgetown, Barbados: E.K. Walters, 1995.

Waterman, I. "A Century of Service". In *The Nursing Council of Trinidad and Tobago Twenty-fifth Anniversary 1950–1975*. Port of Spain, Trinidad: Key Publications, 1975.

Williams, E. *History of the People of Trinidad and Tobago*. Port of Spain, Trinidad: PNM Publishing, 1962.

Video Recordings

Barbados Information Services. *Dame Nita Barrow's Funeral*. Videotape, 20 December 1995.

Jamaica Information Service. *Profiles: Mary Jane Seivwright*. Videotape, 1990.

Index

Adoption: in the West Indies, 139
Adult education: in Jamaica, 24; Nita Barrow in, 55
Advanced Nursing Education Unit (ANEU), xvi, 163–165; aims of, 163; annual evaluation of courses, 166; and fieldwork to Eastern Caribbean, 166–167; follow-up study of graduates, 165–166; and formation of Regional Nursing Body, 193; granted departmental status 171–172; impact of, 164; Mary Seivwright as director of, 160–161, 162; need for accommodation, 165, 167; and Nurse Practitioner Programme, 172–178; objectives of, 165
Alleyne Rawlins, Valerie: on Ben Dolly, 129
Andrewin Staine, Marina: on Mary Seivwright, 162, 181
Annual Nursing Research Conference, 171
Antrobus, Peggy: tribute to Nita Barrow, 65

Baber, Eunice, 124
Bachelor of Science in Nursing, UWI, xvi; approval of proposal for, 169; implementation of, 167–169; introduction of, 169; proposal for, 167
Barbados: public health in, 8–9; social structure of, 10; structure of, 4
Barbados General Hospital: administrative structure of nursing at, 10; nurses training at, 9, 11, 15; patient care at, 10; withholding of nurses certificates, 15
Barrow, Dame Nita, viii, xi, xv, xvi; in adult education, 55; advocacy of improved nurses training, 24; as ambassador to the UN, 60; birth of, 4; bust of, unveiled, 66; and CMC, 48, 51–55; as catalyst in organizing of nurses, 205; characteristics of, 61; in Commonwealth Group of Eminent Persons to South Africa, 57; compared with Ben Dolly and Mary Seivwright, 204–209; as convenor of UN Decade

of Women Conference, 18, 58–59; culinary skills of, 14, 19, 37, 60; death of, 3; in development of Regional Nursing Body, 47; education of, 5–6; experience of racism, 18; as first Caribbean PAHO/WHO nurse, 43; and formation of NAJ, 25; funeral of, 66; as governor general of Barbados, 63–64; and Helen Mussallem, 39; and ICAE, 56–57; at ICN congress, 62–63; international stature of, 57; involvement with YWCA, 48–50; at KPH School of Nursing, 31–32; leadership abilities of, 15–16, 61; as matron of UCHWI, 34; midwifery training of, 17; motivation to enter nursing, 7; on needs of women, 59; as PAHO/WHO nursing advisor, 47; philosophy of, 52; as president of JGTNA, 26, 28; as principal nursing officer of Jamaica, 35–36; public health field experience in Jamaica, 21; and pursuit of bachelor's degree, 38–39; in Registered Nurses' Association, Barbados, 15; as Rockefeller Foundation scholar, 18, 20–21; scholarship to University of Toronto, 18; siblings of, 4; sister tutor's training of, 31; and social justice, 50; and struggle for nurses registration in Jamaica, 114; and survey of nursing schools in the Caribbean, 40, 44–45; training experience of, 12–15; tributes to, 60–62, 63–65; as valedictorian at University of Toronto, 20; and visit to Nelson Mandela, 57–58; and WCC, 48; at WISPH, Jamaica, 21, 22–24

Barrow, Dame Nita, honours and awards: American Jewish Committee award, 18; Caribbean Community's Women's Award, 60–61; CARICOM Triennial Award, 61; Christiane Reimann Award, 62; Dame of the Order of St Andrew and St George, 63; Doctor of Laws, UWI, 50; as West Indian of the Year, 59

Barrow, Reginald, 4–5

Baxter, Ivy, 19

Bayley, Grace, 118

Beckles, Lynne, 89; on Ben Dolly, 112–113, 114

Bishop Anstey High School (Trinidad): impact on Ben Dolly, 87, 99, 100; impact on black girls, 87

Bowen, Hilda: in Regional Nursing Body, 193

Boyd, David, 19

Boyne, Theresa: on Mary Seivwright, 158, 190

Bragg, Lola, 151, 153; on Mary Seivwright, 149

Bragg, Dr Percy, 151

Breaking the Glass Ceiling: choice of title, xvii; expected outcomes of, xi; and health services in the Caribbean, ix; methodology of, xiv–xv

Brome, Dr Rufus: tribute to Nita Barrow, 64–65

Bullen, Nathaniel: and school for black and coloured girls, Barbados, 6

Butler, Uriah, 76

Campbell, Thelma: on Mary Seivwright, 162

Canada: and provision of nurse leaders to Barbados, 16

Caribbean Nursing Organization (CNO), 157; Mary Seivwright and,

Index

192–193; Mavis Harney and, 37–38, 122; objectives of, 122; TTRNA in, 122
Carnegie, M.E., xiv
Carr, Dr Will, 14
Cato, Dr Arnot, 14
Certificated Nurses' Association of Trinidad and Tobago, 106; Ben Dolly in, 107
Champagnie, Leleka, 143, 153, 182, 183, 186; nurses hostel named for, 184
Charles, Dame Eugenia, 19
Chest and Heart Association (Trinidad): Ben Dolly in, 74, 91
Chittick, Dr Rae, 163
Christian Medical Commission (CMC): director's report of Nita Barrow, 53; job of, 51; Nita Barrow and, 48, 51–55; resignation of Nita Barrow from, 54
Cipriani, Arthur, 76
Clapton, R., 124
Class: and education, in Barbados, 5; in Jamaica, 142; and race in nursing, 147; in Trinidad and Tobago, 76
Clyne, Monica, 124
College of Nursing (Trinidad): transfer of nursing education to, 93
Colonial Development and Welfare Fund: and postgraduate training of nurses, 31
Colonialism: and communication barriers in the West Indies, 23
Commission on Higher Education in the Colonies: 24; on a university for the British West Indies, 24; West Indian Committee of, 24
Commonwealth Foundation: and professional centres in Commonwealth countries, 131–132

Commonwealth Nurses Federation: formation of, 128
Commonwealth Nursing Seminar, 207
Communication: colonialism and, in the Caribbean, 23; interisland, 23; independence and, 23
Community nursing care: Ben Dolly on, 104–105
Conference of Caribbean Nursing Administrators: discussions at, 41–42; on regional nursing body, 47; recommendations of, 42; results of, 42; terms of reference of, 41
Coterie of Social Workers: Ben Dolly in, 74, 87; influence of, on Ben Dolly, 86; school feeding programme of, 87
Cotton (Stoute), Nora, 16
Critchlow, Vern, 89

Dame Nita Barrow Award, 57
Darmanie, Ivy, 118
Date Camps, Ada, 89
Dolly, Berenice (Ben), viii, xi, xv, xvi; access of, to opportunities, 78; as administrator of family estate, 90; on being an independent voice, 127; birth of, 97; character of, 132; in Chest and Heart Association (Trinidad), 74, 91; on child rearing, 80–81; children of, 80–85; in church work, 79; at Commonwealth Caribbean nursing conference, 124; on community nursing care, 104–105; compared with Nita Barrow and Mary Seivwright, 204–209; contribution of, described, 130–131; in the Coterie of Social Workers, 74, 87; decision to enter nursing, 99–101; education of, 98–101; and evaluation of Caribbean nursing schools,

125; experience in constitutional matters, 123; family as priority, 85; in formation of Commonwealth Nurses' Federation, 128; on future of professional nursing in Trinidad, 94, 134; goal for nursing, 132; in guiding movement, 99; honoured, 129; on ICN, xv, 115–118; influence of Coterie of Social Workers on, 86; international experiences of, 128; on Julien Commission, 91; on leadership, 92, 107; leadership qualities of, 133; in League of Women Voters, 88–90; on local boards and councils, 92; marriage of, 74–75; nurses training of, 101–104; and Nursing Council of Trinidad and Tobago, 113–114; on nursing education committees, 91, 92–93; parents of, as role models, 98–99; performance in nursing examinations, 103; political involvement of, 88–90; post-basic studies of, 127–128; record keeping skills of, 93; as representative of Western European ideology, 79; as role model, 134; siblings of, 98; in social work, 78–79; in Soroptimist Organization, 90; on specialization in nursing, 79; in Student Nurses' Association, Trinidad, 87, 105–106; and training of local sister tutors, 121; tributes to, 132–133; in TTRNA, 125, 129–132; in Trinidad Orchid Society, 74; in Trinidad and Tobago Agricultural Society, 90; and unification of nursing organizations in Trinidad, 106–107, 205; value of social contacts of, 93; views of, on male position in the household, 77–78; views of, on married nursing students, 104; in volunteer work, 74, 78

Dolly, Berenice, honours and awards: Business and Professional Women's Club award, 92; Coterie of Social Workers' Distinguished Service Award, 87; Distinguished Service Awards, TTRNA, 131; Medal of Merit (Gold), Order of the Trinity, 92; OBE, 86; San Fernando Borough Council award, 92; Soroptimist service award, 90; as *Trinidad Guardian* distinguished "75er", 94; Trinidad and Tobago Alliance of the USA award, 132

Dolly, Hilary: on Ben Dolly, 82–84; on relationship between parents, 85

Dolly, Dr Reynold, 77; death of, 84; marriage of, to Ben Dolly, 74–75

Dolly, Stephen: on Ben Dolly, 82

Dolly-Hargreaves Building, 115

Duke, Beulah: on Mary Seivwright, 194

Education: and class, in Barbados, 5; of girls, in Barbados, 5; and social mobility, 140, 142

Esteen, Pearlie: on Mary Seivwright, 181, 182

Federation, West Indian, 29; and regional cooperation in nursing, 41, 122, 123, 157

Feminism: in nursing, 27

Fields, Lucy, 121, 122

Flash O'Sullivan, Lucy, 152, 186; on Mary Seivwright, 178–179

Foster, Valerie, 121, 122; on Mary Seivwright, 194

Francis, Dr Aldwyn, 111

Index

Fraser, Carmeta: tribute to Nita Barrow, 61–62

Freedom of movement: for nurses in the Caribbean, 36

Fuller, Enid, 146

Garvey, Marcus, 141; and UNIA, 141

Gender-role stereotyping: in middle class Trinidad, 81–82

General Nursing Council for England and Wales: and entrance examinations in Britain, 120; administration of entrance test in Trinidad, 121; and recognition of nurses' training, 42

Gibbs, Revd Luther, 143

Gibson, Eunice, 17

Gillette, Dr Horace, 41, 111, 124

Grant, James Emmanuel: as father of Ben Dolly, 97, 100; and Pharmaceutical Society of Trinidad and Tobago, 97

Grant, Mary: on Mary Seivwright, 170–171

Grassfield School (Barbados), 6

Grayson, Dr Jean: and 3M International Award, 129–130; on Ben Dolly, 130, 132

Griffith, Eunice, 15

Hanson, Merel: as ICN vice president, 185; on Mary Seivwright, 181, 185, 188–189

Harding, Marion, 124

Harney, Mavis: and CNO, 37–38, 122

Haslam, Phyllis, 48

Health for All by the Year 2000, 51

Health initiatives: in the Caribbean, 1940s and 1950s, 24

Henderson, Virginia

Hewitt, Hermi: on Mary Seivwright, 179

Hine, D.C., xiii

Hospitals: Barbados General Hospital, 9–11; Kingston Public Hospital (Jamaica), 31; St James General Hospital (Jamaica), 146; staffing of, in Trinidad, 102–103

Huffman (Splane), Verna, 42

Independence: and interisland communication, 23

Insularity: of Jamaica, 23

International Alliance of Women: Ben Dolly in, 128

International Council of Adult Education (ICAE), 55; and Dame Nita Barrow Award, 57; management structure of, 56–57; Nita Barrow and, 56; Roby Kidd and, 55; women and the work of, 56

International Council of Nurses (ICN), xv; award to Nita Barrow, 62; Ben Dolly on, xv, 115–118; benefits of membership in, 118; Jamaica and Trinidad as members of, 205; Mary Seivwright and, 158–160, 196; TNMATT membership on, 116–117

Jackson, D. Hamilton, 4

Jacobs, Ann, 34, 35

Jamaica: brief background of, 140–142; class in, 142; economic stratification by race, 141; as hub of West Indian healthcare activities, 29; independence of, 141; insularity of, 23; peasantry of, 141; political system of, in 1930s, 141; riots, in 1938; 141; school system of, in 1920s and 30s, 142–143; social conditions, 21; social stratification in, 141–142; universal adult suffrage, 141

219

Jamaica Civil Service Association: and representation of nurses, 185–186

Jamaica General Trained Nurses Association (JGTNA): formation of, 26, 148; goals of, 26; headquarters of, 28. *See also* Nurses Association of Jamaica (NAJ)

Jamaica Welfare Ltd.: adult education programme of, 24

Jeffers, Audrey, 7, 74; and Coterie of Social Workers, 86; influence of, on Ben Dolly, 86–87; as role model for black women in Trinidad, 86

Joseph, Roy, 111; and nurses registration bill, Trinidad, 111–112

Julien Commission (Trinidad), 91; Ben Dolly on, 120; findings of, 120–121; terms of reference of, 120

Kidd, Roby: and ICAE, 55
Kingston Public Hospital (Jamaica), 31; School of Nursing at, 31–32

'Lady' boats, 17, 18
Landsberg, Michele, 60; remembrance of Nita Barrow, 60
Lawrence, Enid, 171, 182; as director of Nurse Practitioner Programme, 176–177
Lawrence, Ivy, 19
Leadership: abilities of Nita Barrow, 15–16, 61; Ben Dolly on, 92, 107; lack of, in nursing in Jamaica, 147; Mary Seivwright and, 161; qualities of Ben Dolly, 133
League of Women Voters (Trinidad): Ben Dolly in, 128; founding of, 88. *See also* National League of Women Voters

Lightbourne, Dr Hyacinth: and support for nurses' registration in Jamaica, 27
Lowe, Eva, 124
Lumsden, Ann, 100
Lusan, Carmen, 28, 49; on characteristics of Nita Barrow, 61

MacGilvray, Dr James, 51
MacManus, Emily, 26, 110, 147; report of, on nurses training in the West-Indies, 147–148. *See also* MacManus Nursing Commission
MacManus Nursing Commission, 110, 147–148. s*See also* MacManus, Emily
Mandela, Nelson: visit of Nita Barrow to, 57–58
Marshall-Burnett, Syringa: on Mary Seacole, xiv; on Mary Seivwright, 171
Mary Seivwright Day, 139, 171
Massiah, Joan: on Ben Dolly, 81; on racial discrimination at Pointe-à-Pierre, Trinidad, 84
Masson, Jessie, 106
Matthews, Marie, 47
McLean, Helen, 36
McShine, Leonora: and League of Women Voters, Trinidad, 88
Medical Board ordinance: and control of nursing in Trinidad, 97
Metivier, Avis, 99, 106; and agitation for advancement of nurses in Trinidad, 103
Midwifery training: in Trinidad, 17, 102
Midwives: status of, in Trinidad, 102
Mitchell, Irene, 133
Montenegro, Irene, 118, 133; on Ben Dolly, 119
Morgan, Peter: tribute to Nita Barrow, 63

Moyne Commission: findings in Trinidad and Tobago, 76; on public health in the West Indies, 12, 147; results of, 31
Murray Ainsley, Ilene, 13, 22
Mussallem, Helen: and Nita Barrow, 39, 60

National Institute for Higher Education, Research, Science and Technology (NIHERST) (Trinidad), 93
National League of Women Voters (Trinidad): activities of, 89; objectives of, 88–89. *See also* League of Women Voters
Nightengale Nurses' Home: building of, in Barbados, 14; 33n. 8
Nightingale, Florence, xiii
Nurse anaesthetists: registration of, in Jamaica, 191
Nurse leaders, viii, xiii; changes in, in Canada, 16
Nurse practitioners: qualifications and responsibilities, 175–176
Nurse Practitioner Programme, xvi, 172–178; administrative difficulties of, 176; continuing education component of, 177; Enid Lawrence as director of, 176–177; Joint Nurse Practitioner Advisory Committee, 176; NAJ and introduction of, 174, 188; outlined, 175; Project HOPE and, 174; protocol manual for, 178, 202n. 13; Winston Davidson and, 174–175
Nurses: accomplishments of Caribbean, x; Caribbean, in nursing history, xiv; group training of, at Barbados General Hospital, 11; migration of, from Jamaica, 185; opportunities for advancement, in Jamaica, 147; and perceptions of nursing, 105; political awakening of, in Barbados, 9; renewal of licences, in Jamaica, 191; working conditions of, in Jamaica, 26, 185
Nurses' Association of Jamaica (NAJ), xvi; accommodation for, 183–184; constitutional changes, 188; contribution of Mary Seivwright to, 181–185; credit union of, 183; history of, 25–29; and introduction of Nurse Practitioner Programme, 174, 188; manual of, 183; membership drive of, 186; Nita Barrow and, 25; as nurses' bargaining unit, 185–186, 188; and nurses' housing, 184; position paper on nursing in Jamaica, 182; recognition of contribution of Mary Sievwright, 188
Nurses, black, x, xiv
Nurses exchange programme: in Jamaica, 149
Nurses and Midwives Registration Act, Barbados, 9
Nurses Ordinance (Trinidad), 97
Nurses organizations: formation of, in Trinidad, 106
Nurses' Registration Ordinance No. 38 (Trinidad): passage of, 112
Nurses training: apprenticeship system of, 11, 147, 205; block system of, 109, 135n. 5; decentralization of, in Jamaica, 146; deficiencies in basic, 24; deterioration in, in Trinidad, 101; group training at Barbados General Hospital, 11; male physicians in, 147; need for revision of, in Trinidad, 101; in Trinidad, 102; physicians' role in,

in Jamaica, 146; reforms in, in Jamaica, 146

Nursing: agitation for principal nursing officer in Jamaica, 35; feminism in, 27; gender and power bias in, 191–192; hidden heroines of Caribbean, 208; influences on, in 1930s Barbados, 10–11; lack of leadership in, in Jamaica, 147; married women and, 104; perceptions of, in early 20th century Jamaica, 145; race and class and, 147; regionalism and, 206

Nursing Council (Barbados): formation of, 9; and training of nurses, 9–10

Nursing Council (Jamaica), xvi; contribution of Mary Seivwright to, 189; establishment of, 28; and evaluation of nursing schools, 190

Nursing Council of Trinidad and Tobago: establishment of, 112; interim, 113; and registration of midwives, 114–115; responsibilities of, 113

Nursing education: advanced programme recommended, 46; need to preserve indigenous practices and traditions in, 94; reciprocity of, in the Caribbean region, 36; reforms in, in Jamaica, 146; Seminar, 1968, 163; standard of, in the Caribbean, 24; standard of, in Trinidad, 130; University of Toronto and, 16. *See also* ANEU

Nursing schools. *See* Schools of Nursing

Nutting, Adelaide, xiii

O'Neal, Dr Duncan: community activism of, 6–7; political leadership of, 7

O'Neal, Ebenezer, 17

Page, Mary, 9

PAHO/WHO: and advanced nursing education programmes, 163; Nursing Education Seminar, 1971, ix; and survey of nursing schools in the Caribbean, 40, 43

Patient care: stratification of, at Barbados General Hospital, 10

Peters, Pearl, 112, 118

Pharmaceutical Society of Trinidad and Tobago, 97

Pilgrim, Yvonne, 92; on Ben Dolly, 129

Port of Spain Trained Nurses' Association, 106

Port of Spain Trained Nurses and Midwives Association, 106

Potter, Philip, 51; tribute to Nita Barrow, 65

Principal nursing officer: agitation for, in Jamaica, 35

Professional centres: built, in Trinidad, 132; establishment of, in Commonwealth countries, 132

Professions: availability of, to women in Barbados, 8

Project HOPE, 201n. 11; and nurse practitioner programme, 174

Public health: conditions in Jamaica, in the 1930s, 145–146

Public Health Commission: appointment of, in Barbados, 9; recommendations of, in Barbados, 9

Public health nursing: course at University of Toronto, 16; need for training in the Caribbean, 19

Purvis, Nancy: contribution to nurses training in Barbados, 12

Racism: in Barbados, 5, 15; Nita Barrow's experience of, 18

Ramphal, Sir Shridath: on Nita Barrow's visit to Nelson Mandela, 57–58
Regional Nursing Body: advocated, 122, 170; ANEU and formation of, 193; formed, 159; recommendation on nursing education, 168; recommended by Conference of Caribbean Nursing Administrators, 47
Regionalism: and nursing in the Caribbean, 206
Registered Nurses' Association (Barbados), 15s
Registration of nurses: in Barbados, 7–8, 9; benefits of, 27, 29; government committee to examine, in Trinidad, 111; in Jamaica, 26–28, 149, 205; pursuit of, in Trinidad, 108–112, 114, 205; in Trinidad, 102
Rigsby, Lorna, 80; on Ben Dolly, 85
Ristori, Isabella, 105–106, 116; and agitation for advancement of nurses in Trinidad, 103
Robb, Isabel, xiii
Rockefeller Foundation: and support of post-basic nursing education, 16, 17
Rushcliffe Committee: recommendations of, 109, 147; work of, 147

St James General Hospital (Jamaica), 146
San Fernando Study Group (Trinidad): formation of, 88
Schools of Nursing: administration, conduct and evaluation of survey of, 43–47; in Kingston, Jamaica, 146; minimum uniform standards for, in Jamaica, 190; need for survey of West Indian, 39; resurvey of, requested, 47–48; survey of, in the Caribbean, viii, 157; survey recommended, for the Caribbean, 42, 124–125; recommendations of the survey of, 46–47
Science: lack of teaching, for girls in Trinidad, 121
Scrub nurse, 33n. 9
Seacole, Mary, xiv
Sealy, Ivy, 7
Sealy, Dr Karen, 61
Seivwright, Dr Mary, viii, ix, xi, xv, xvi; acceptance for nurses' training, 145; achievement in nursing training, 148; as activist, 192–194; administrative style of, 170–171; as administrator and researcher, 165–171; and advocacy of Faculty of Health Sciences at UWI, 172; beliefs of, 157–158; birth of, 139; bypassing of, for promotion, 150–152; in Caribbean nursing education, 194; and change of NAJ's constitution, 188; as chief project nurse, 156; choice of nursing as career, 144–145; at CNO meetings, 157, 192; commitment to nursing research, 178; at Commonwealth Caribbean Nurses Meeting, Barbados, 159; compared with Ben Dolly and Nita Barrow, 204–209; contribution to NAJ, 181–185; contribution to Nursing Council of Jamaica, 189–192; as Dean's Scholar, 156; and development of Nurse Practitioner Programme, 173–178; and development of vena puncture policy, 190–191; and differences with colonial administrators, 151–152; as director of ANEU, 160–161, 162; early education of, 143–144; excellence as mission of, 156; as feminist, 179, 196; and follow-up study of ANEU

223

graduates, 166–167; and formation of NAJ's credit union, 183; at Francis Delafield Hospital, 150, 153; goal of, 164; at Hebrew Hospital for the Chronic Sick, USA, 156; and ICN, 158–160, 196; impact on socioeconomic conditions of nurses, 185–186, 188; and implementation of BSc Nursing degree, 167–169; in leadership position in Jamaica, 161; love of gardening, 143, 199; on Mary Seacole, xiv; midwifery training of, 148; as NAJ president, 181; in nursing research in Jamaica, 154–155; as nursing research project director, 154–155; and opening address of NAJ summer school, 1967, 157; philosophy of, 158; policy making experience of, 180; political involvement of, 195–196; as President's Scholar, 150, 153; as public health nurse, 148–153; and pursuit of BSc nursing degree, 149, 150; and pursuit of Ed. D degree, 155; and pursuit of Master's degree, 153; in Regional Nursing Body, 193; and religion, 200; and renewal of nurses' licences, 191; research on youth and nursing, 191–192; resignation from Nursing Council of Jamaica, 192; responsibilities of, as chief project nurse, 156; retirement of, 197–198; as senator, 195–197; sense of nationalism of, 142; siblings of, 139; as teacher and mentor, 178–181; teaching style of, 179–180; triple first in training, 148; on value of nursing research, 198; visit to Nurses' Association of Dominica, 159–160; at Visiting Nurse Services of New York, 149–150; at WISPH, 148–149

Seivwright, Mary, honours and awards: for community service (Jaycees), 178; Doctor of Humanities degree, 198; naming of Mary Jane Seivwright building, 198; Nursing Education Alumni Association award, 169; Order of Distinction, Jamaica, 164; Order of Jamaica, 192, 198; Woman of Distinction award, 197

Sexism: in Barbados, 5

Shenton, Blanche, 26, 110, 147

Simmons, Dr Leo W., 154

Simmons, Sybil, 7

Sister tutors: need for, identified, 148; recruitment of tutor for Barbados, 9; training of local, in Trinidad, 121

Social mobility: education and, 140, 142

Social networks: value of, 93, 113

Soroptimist Organization: Ben Dolly in, 128; purpose of, 90

South Certificated Nurses' Association, 106. *See also* Certificated Nurses' Association of Trinidad and Tobago

Standard (Francis), Evelyn, 34, 66

Standard, Sir Kenneth: on Mary Seivwright, 170

Stevens, May, 124

Swaby, Gertrude, 32, 182

Symes, Julie, 182

Teaching: and black women in early 20th century, 144

Thomas (Wolfe), Mary, 21, 22

Thompson, Janet, 36, 41, 42, 47

Thompson, Fr Robert: on Mary Seivwright, 200

Thorne, Grace, 7

Trained Nurses and Midwives' Association of Trinidad and Tobago (TNMATT): and nursing education in Trinidad, 111; name change of, 114; and nursing scholarships, 109–110; work of the unified association, 107–108; formation of, 107

Travel: interisland, in the 1940s, 17

Trinidad Counselling and Advisory Service (TRINCAS): formation of, 125; functions of, 125–126

Trinidad Guardian: selection of Ben Dolly as distinguished "75er", 94

Trinidad and Tobago: abolition of indentureship in; 76; adult franchise in, 76; brief history of, 75–77; class distinction in, 76; independence of, 77; rise of labour movement in, 76; socioeconomic condition in, 1930s and 1940s, 76; oil in, 76

Trinidad and Tobago Agricultural Society: Ben Dolly in, 90

Trinidad and Tobago Registered Nurses' Association (TTRNA), 92, 114; in CNO, 122; counselling programme of, 125; and Extra-Mural Department (UWI) courses, 121; and pre-nursing scholarships, 120; and refresher courses, 119–120; tribute to Ben Dolly, 132

Udell, Florence, 35

UN Decade of Women Conference: Nita Barrow as convenor of, 58–59

Universal Negro Improvement Association (UNIA): and black working class activists, 141

University College Hospital of the West Indies (UCHWI), 24; as impetus for improvements in nursing education, 32; and interisland communication, 23; opening of, 34; West Indian nursing staff at, 32

University Hospital of the West Indies. *See* UCHWI

University of Toronto: and nursing education, 16; public health nursing course at, 16; West Indian students at, 19–20

Vena puncture: NAJ policy on, 190–191

Walls, Marion, 107

Walters, Ena, 47, 124; and Regional Nursing Body, 193

Walton, Alice, 145, 146; and reforms in nursing education, Jamaica, 146

Waterman, Ivy, 106, 111, 113

Waterman, Dr James, 111

West Indian students: at University of Toronto, 19–20

West Indies School of Public Health (WISPH), 109; establishment of, 23, 24; Nita Barrow at, 22–24; post-diploma nursing programme at, 23

Women: in the Caribbean, in colonial era, 204; options open to, in the colonial Caribbean, 204; professions open to black, in Barbados, 8; role of Caribbean, 195; and search for recognition, 59; and work of ICAE, 56

World Council of Churches (WCC): Nita Barrow and, 48, 50; work of, 50

Young Reid, Yvonne: on Mary Seivwright, 179

YWCA: Nita Barrow as president of World YWCA, 48–50

ISBN 141201517-0